Maharishi Mahesh Yogi's

TRANSCENDENTAL MEDITATION

Maharishi Mahesh Yogi's

TM

TRANSCENDENTAL MEDITATION

Revised & Updated Edition

A New Introduction to Maharishi's Easy, Effective and Scientifically Proven Technique for Promoting Better Health, Unfolding Your Creative Potential— and Creating Peace in the World

by Robert Roth

Primus

DONALD I. FINE, INC.
NEW YORK

Library of Congress Catalogue Card Number: 94-071116
ISBN: 1-55611-403-6
Manufactured in the United States of America
10 9 8 7 6 5 4 3 2

Printed in the United States of America

"My practice of Transcendental Meditation has given me a 360-degree awareness. In business, I have always been very fixed and focused on my goals, and now, with the expanded awareness gained from Transcendental Meditation, I am able to be more open and flexible in my approaches to achieving these goals. In my personal life, I feel that I am a far more integrated, fulfilled human being."

—Tom Gould, Chairman and CEO, Younkers, Inc., a chain of 53 fashion-department stores throughout the Midwest. Mr. Gould has been practicing Transcendental Meditation for 7 years.

"I have two full-time jobs. I am the mother of two children and I am a doctor. For me personally, Transcendental Meditation is like taking a vacation twice a day. After a long day at the office or teaching medical students at the Erie County Medical Center, I feel completely refreshed and revitalized after Transcendental Meditation. I can't imagine how people live without it."

—Margaret Mitchell, M.D., a specialist in geriatrics, Buffalo, New York. Dr. Mitchell has been practicing Transcendental Meditation for 16 years.

"**Transcendental Meditation allows my mind to** completely settle down for 20 minutes, and I find that extremely refreshing. As a result, I am able to do my job better with less stress. I am able to stay calm under pressure in a world of uncalm people. The technique lends clarity to my thinking and allows me to prioritize better and know where to put my energy and focus."

—Judy Garvey, Principal of Easterbrook School, San Jose, California. Ms. Garvey has been practicing Transcendental Meditation for 18 years.

"**I feel closer to myself; I know myself better. I am** more sensitive to my own feelings and desires, and I know more clearly what is right and wrong for me. Actually, I believe that everyone knows what is right and wrong, but it is clouded over by stress. Transcendental Meditation has allowed me to read those signs very quickly and clearly."

—Sam Lieb, first-year theater major, Northwestern University, Evanston, Illinois. Sam has been practicing Transcendental Meditation for 8 years.

"I have sat on the divorce court in Chicago for 12 years. Stress has been a given in my everyday life; I have been inundated by it.

"I turned to Transcendental Meditation in an effort to reduce stress and draw on resources of peace and serenity. The first thing I noticed was that I shed a burden of fatigue. And even though I have achieved a lot in my life, I have also been quite a procrastinator. From the very first day, I experienced that I had the energy and enthusiasm for tasks that had eluded me. But something more has happened. I have found a subtle, but very real, enhancement of my clarity. I now perceive things around me with greater sharpness of mind. I spend my life as a trained observer, so this has been a very valuable result.

"My professional life is led in very serious terms; so much so that I used to find that I wasn't able to laugh enough or enjoy myself in my personal life. Since starting Transcendental Meditation, I find that I am spontaneously laughing much more with my family and friends. I learned the technique as a way to manage stress. What I have gotten is more than I ever expected. Transcendental Meditation has enhanced so many facets of my life. I am surprised and very pleased."

—The Hon. Susan Snow, Associate Judge, Circuit Court of Cook County, Illinois, Domestic Relations Division. Judge Snow has been practicing Transcendental Meditation for 3 weeks.

"I find that the two 20-minute periods of Transcendental Meditation give me inner calm, great energy, and far more presence of mind with which to serve the people of God. Transcendental Meditation involves no faith or belief and may be practiced with confidence by any religious person."

—Father Kevin Joyce, Pastor of the St. Maria Goretti Church in San Jose, California, a large multicultural and multilingual parish. Father Joyce has been practicing Transcendental Meditation for over 20 years.

"Being a new mom is one of the most wonderful experiences I've ever had. But as everyone knows, not getting enough rest can be a big problem. So for me to be able to sit down for 20 minutes twice a day and get that deep rest from Transcendental Meditation makes a tremendous difference, especially when I'm getting up several times during the night. I feel very relaxed, and I think that comes out in Lucas. He's a wonderful baby, content and always happy. I credit Transcendental Meditation for having such a positive influence in our family life."

—Christine Reed, Chapel Hill, North Carolina. Mrs. Reed is the mother of a two-month-old baby boy, Lucas. She has been practicing Transcendental Meditation for 11 years.

"A little over a year ago I was diagnosed with multiple sclerosis. It came as a complete shock to me because I had just gone through 10 years of training to become a physician. I was encouraged to cut back on my workload so I could get enough rest. I spoke with some MS experts about different options available to deal with the disorder. As it's been well-documented that stress makes MS worse and adds to the disease process, I chose to learn Transcendental Meditation. I've been meditating for 5 months now, and I feel better than I've felt in 10 years. I'm actually working more hours today than I was before the diagnosis. Transcendental Meditation has helped me in a multitude of other ways. It's helped me professionally, as it would any physician who has to deal with constant stress, and it's helped me personally in my relationships and in promoting my own good health."

—Patricia Ammon, M.D., family practice, Ouray, Colorado. Dr. Ammon has been practicing Transcendental Meditation for 5 months.

Table of Contents

Author's Note

Something dramatic is happening in America. Just about everyone in the nation is waking up to a very simple, profound fact: *Prevention is always better than cure*. Chronic fatigue, anxiety, high blood pressure, heart disease, many forms of cancer, even crime and violence are far more effectively and cost-effectively prevented than they are treated or cured.

And something else is happening, too. In the 7 years since *Maharishi Mahesh Yogi's Transcendental Meditation* was first published, more and more doctors and other health care professionals, business and community leaders, educators, and members of the general public have come to appreciate the enormous practical benefits of Transcendental Meditation. They are endorsing the use of this simple technique in prevention-oriented programs to reduce stress and disease, improve health, reduce crime and violence, and improve the quality of life for the individual and society.

The old saying is a wise one: "There is nothing more powerful than an idea whose time has come." Transcendental Meditation is much more than an idea—it is a powerful, proven technology to unfold our most precious natural resource—the human mind. It is a technology whose time has come. The whole of society is already the better for it—the future will be even brighter.

—*Robert Roth*

1

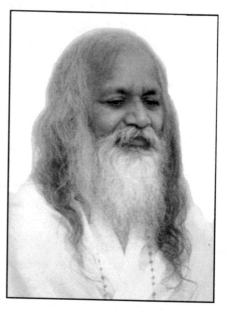

MAHARISHI MAHESH YOGI

Founder of the
Transcendental Meditation
and TM-Sidhi Program
Maharishi Vedic Universities
Maharishi Ayur Veda Universities
Maharishi International University

Introduction

On January 29, 1959, Maharishi Mahesh Yogi arrived at San Francisco International Airport. It was his first visit to the United States, and the second continent on his global tour to introduce his Transcendental Meditation technique to the world.

Maharishi lectured to hundreds of people during his 2-month stay; many people learned the technique. The *San Francisco Chronicle* covered one of Maharishi's lectures and published the first article on Transcendental Meditation ever in America.

Maharishi's message then was simple and direct, and it's the same today. Life is bliss. Man is born to enjoy. Within everyone is an unlimited reservoir of energy, intelligence, and happiness. Transcendental Meditation is a simple, effortless procedure to experience it. The technique can be easily learned by anyone of any age, culture, religion, or educational background.

In those early days, there were no other Transcendental Meditation teachers, no Transcendental Meditation centers. After San Francisco, Maharishi spent several months in Los Angeles, then traveled on to New York. From New York, Maharishi went to England, Germany, Greece, and on around the world.

The Transcendental Meditation movement started simply and grew steadily. Then suddenly, with the first published scientific research on the technique, Transcendental Meditation gained worldwide recognition.

The first study on Maharishi's Transcendental Meditation was conducted at the University of California at Los Angeles in 1968 by physiologist Robert Keith Wallace. His thesis, "The Physiological Effects of Transcendental Meditation: A Proposed Fourth Major State of Consciousness," earned him his Ph.D., and his findings were published in the journals *Science* and *Scientific American*. This also inspired a huge upsurge of research into the effects of Transcendental Meditation.

By 1975 Transcendental Meditation was a household word.

And today? More than four million people worldwide—including more than one million people in the United States—from every profession, age, educational background, and religion practice Transcendental Meditation. And the number keeps growing.

The technique has been learned by over 6,000 medical doctors in the U.S. and by tens of thousands of executives, managers, and employees of large corporations and small businesses throughout the U.S. and the world.

Homemakers practice Transcendental Meditation. So do attorneys, computer programmers, teachers, students, sales clerks, clergy, athletes, factory workers, architects, airline pilots, electricians, chefs, and artists.

Why? Transcendental Meditation is easy to learn. Anyone can practice it. And it works.

During the past 25 years, more than 500 scientific research studies have been conducted on the effects of the Transcendental Meditation technique at 210 independent universities and research institutions in 33 countries. The studies—many of which have been published in leading scientific journals—have shown that the Transcendental Meditation program:

- Reduces stress
- Increases creativity and intelligence
- Improves memory and learning ability
- Increases energy
- Increases inner calm
- Reduces insomnia
- Increases happiness and self-esteem
- Reduces anxiety and depression
- Improves relationships
- Improves health
- Promotes a younger biological age.

Since Maharishi first began teaching the Transcendental Meditation technique over 36 years ago, modern science has made major breakthroughs in understanding how nature functions. Recently, scientists have glimpsed the deepest level of nature's functioning—the unified field of natural law—which is the source of the unlimited creative potential displayed throughout the universe.

As we'll see in this book, the unlimited potential found deep within human consciousness and the unlimited potential found at the level of the unified field are not different; they are the same.

Transcendental Meditation is a simple, effective technique that enlivens the unlimited potential of life from its source in the unified field. It enriches all areas of life, just as watering the root of a plant brings nourishment to all parts of the plant.

This book has been written to provide you with a brief and complete introduction to the Transcendental Meditation program. It is an introduction to the technique that can change your life for good.

I hope you enjoy it.

CHAPTER 1

Transcendental Meditation at a Glance

A Harvard graduate student asked his instructor, Ronald David, M.D., about meditation. What was it? What did it do? Dr. David, Lecturer in Public Policy at the John F. Kennedy School of Government, offered to find out. He called the Transcendental Meditation Center in Cambridge, and the next week a speaker addressed Dr. David's class. Fascinated, six students, along with Dr. David, started the technique.

It's now 18 months later, 8:00 a.m. on a Tuesday—one of the busiest days of the week for Dr. David. He sits in his office, notes for today's lectures piled on his desk. But before he starts to review them—and before his office turns busy—he turns off the ringer on his telephone, closes his eyes, and begins his morning practice of Transcendental Meditation.

"I finish meditating and I start the day feeling alert, creative, energized, and much more organized," Dr. David says.

Later that morning, after going over his notes with

a colleague, Dr. David, a noted pediatrician-turned-policy analyst, will lecture to 42 graduate students on "Risk and Resilience in Childhood: Implications for Public Policy." After lunch, he will make final preparations for, and then teach, a 3-hour afternoon seminar.

"At the end of what has normally been a hectic pace and before I get on the train to go home, I close the door to my office, again turn off the ringer on the telephone, and meditate. I wind down from the tension of the day; it leaves me completely refreshed and alert for the train ride back, so I can do something I enjoy, such as read a book, rather than just fall asleep."

As a health policy analyst, Dr. David sees significant applications for Transcendental Meditation.

"We have focused too long and too exclusively on the medical model of management," Dr. David says. "I am impressed with the emerging data on the role of Transcendental Meditation in the treatment of intractable hypertension, reduction of recidivism in prison inmates, and recovery from drug addiction—particularly among African Americans.

"For me Transcendental Meditation is much more profound than simply a physiological way of relaxing. It's a way of becoming whole, of experiencing our own deep inner connectedness as human beings. That experience gives a far greater capacity for health and healing."

What exactly is Transcendental Meditation?
And what is it not?
What are the benefits? How does it work?
The first thing to know about the Transcendental Meditation program of Maharishi Mahesh Yogi is that it's easy to learn and enjoyable to practice.

Second, scientific research shows that the benefits of Transcendental Meditation can be seen immediately and accumulate over time.

Third, it's simple to understand.

What Transcendental Meditation Is
Transcendental Meditation is a simple, natural, effortless, easily-learned mental technique practiced for 15 to 20 minutes twice daily, sitting comfortably with the eyes closed.

To elaborate:

• **Simple**—Transcendental Meditation is *not* difficult or complicated; it is a simple procedure.

• **Natural**—there is no manipulation or suggestion, such as in hypnosis.

• **Effortless**—Transcendental Meditation is easy to practice and requires no ability to concentrate or control the mind.

• **Easily learned**—anyone beginning from age 10 can learn Transcendental Meditation easily.

• **Mental technique**—it requires no physical exercises, special postures, or procedures.

• **Practiced for 15 to 20 minutes twice daily**—Transcendental Meditation is practiced for 15 to 20 minutes: once in the morning before breakfast, to start the day with alertness and energy, and once again in the afternoon before dinner, to eliminate the accumulated stress of the day and as a basis for an enjoyable evening and a good night's sleep.

• **Sitting comfortably**—no awkward or cramped positions are necessary to practice Transcendental Meditation. You can practice the technique anywhere—in your office after work, riding the subway, sitting in a plane, or even in your car parked at a highway rest stop. But it is usually practiced in the comfort of your own home.

What Happens During Transcendental Meditation

During Transcendental Meditation the mind settles down to a silent, yet fully awake, state of awareness—pure consciousness. At the same time the body gains a unique and profound state of rest and relaxation.

To understand the experience of the mind and body settling down during Transcendental Meditation, we'll take two common occurrences.

Excited mind: It's Friday, 2:00 p.m. It's been a busy day and a long week. You're late for an appointment. You race to your car only to realize that you've forgotten your keys. You find your keys, and then you have to battle traffic and road construction before finally making it to your appointment—only to discover that you've left behind some important papers. Your mind is speeding, and your heart is pounding.

Settled mind: It's Sunday afternoon and you're heading home from a long weekend vacation, rested and refreshed. You feel contented, relaxed, happy. Your mind is alert, calm, clear. You begin to think of new ways to make things better at work and at home—good, practical ideas.

Both of these experiences—of greater and of lesser excitation of mind and body—are already very familiar to us.

Now what does Transcendental Meditation do?

Transcendental Meditation is a systematic technique that allows mental activity to settle down to a silent state of awareness where the mind is calm, collected, yet fully expanded, fully awake.

This state is the simplest form of human awareness. It is pure consciousness, a state of "self-referral" awareness open only to itself—open to its own full potential. And as we'll see in the next chapter, it is the unified field of natural law, which modern physics describes as the source of the infinite creativity and intelligence of nature.

This settled state is completely natural to the mind. It has always been there. It was there 10 years ago, it's there right now, and it'll be there tomorrow. Only it has been lost from experience, lost from use, because of the constant noise and pressures and excitations of daily life.

Transcendental Meditation allows the mind to

experience pure consciousness easily, effortlessly, and enjoyably. At the same time, extensive scientific research has shown that while the mind settles down during Transcendental Meditation, the body gains a state of profound rest and relaxation that is far deeper than any other technique of meditation or relaxation produces.

Benefits of Transcendental Meditation

What are the benefits of this experience?

Pure consciousness is the source of the unlimited creativity and intelligence of the mind. Research has shown that the twice daily experience of pure consciousness during Transcendental Meditation makes the mind more alert, creative, and intelligent throughout the day.

And the deep rest provided by Transcendental Meditation eliminates the build-up of stress and tension; improves health; and provides the basis for more dynamic, productive, and satisfying activity.

Not All Rest Is Equal

Rest eliminates stress. The deeper the rest, the better. The rest gained during a night's sleep is sufficient to eliminate some of the stress and fatigue that comes from a full day of activity. But obviously a night's sleep, no matter how deep, isn't enough. We may feel better the next morning, but all too often we don't feel completely refreshed, completely free from the fatigue of the day—and days—before.

So we may exercise to help cope with stress—play tennis, work out at the gym, take an evening walk—or listen to music, read a book, knit a sweater, or go on a fishing trip.

But something is missing. Despite our best efforts, stress clings to the nervous system and builds up day after day, year after year. Butterflies in the stomach from pre-exam nerves at age 16 can turn into stomach ulcers, high blood pressure, or premature aging, at age 40—all from too many years of too much worry.

What is missing? Very, very deep rest.

Recreation or a vacation may be relaxing, but they don't provide the depth of rest necessary to eliminate accumulated stress. Because of this, the benefits are short-lived. (Recall your first day back at work after a week-long vacation. Within a few hours it feels like you never left.)

What is the solution?

Deep Rest Eliminates Deep Stress

Transcendental Meditation. It provides very deep rest—which is exactly what the body needs to eliminate the very deeply-rooted stress that sleep or a vacation never touch.

In one stroke of Transcendental Meditation, the mind and body are rejuvenated. Then you can play tennis, work in the garden, read a book, or go fishing, because you enjoy it, and not because you are trying to cope with an ever-increasing amount of stress in life.

All Techniques Are Not the Same

Are all meditation and relaxation techniques the same? Are all their benefits equal?

No. Four major "meta-analyses" have been published that compare findings of hundreds of scientific studies on Transcendental Meditation and all other forms of meditation and relaxation. The studies show clearly that Transcendental Meditation is far more effective in reducing anxiety; improving psychological health; increasing self-actualization; and reducing cigarette, drug, and alcohol misuse.

Practical Technique for
Health, Happiness, and Success

For a long, long time meditation has been considered the domain of recluses. For people with families and jobs, meditation, at its best, was seen as a momentary refuge from the demands of living; at its worst, an escape from life.

Transcendental Meditation is neither. It is a practical, proven technique for developing more energy, creativity, and intelligence—for awakening the unlimited potential of mind and body and enjoying greater health, happiness, and success in life.

What Transcendental Meditation Is Not

Transcendental Meditation is not a religion, a philosophy, or a lifestyle. Nor does it involve any codes of conduct or moral training, a value system, belief, or worship. To elaborate:

- **Transcendental Meditation is not a religion—** it's a technique. Millions of people of all religions, including clergy, practice Transcendental Meditation. It supports all religions because it releases stress and purifies the mind, body, and emotions of the person who practices it.

- **Transcendental Meditation is not a philosophy—** it's a simple, mechanical technique. Turning on a light switch is a technique; it involves no philosophy. Using a lever to move a large rock is a technique; it involves no philosophy. And Transcendental Meditation is a scientific technique because it is universally applicable, repeatable, and verifiable by anyone, anywhere.

- **Transcendental Meditation is not a lifestyle—** it's a technique. You don't have to change your lifestyle in order to start Transcendental Meditation. Just learn it, practice it, and enjoy the benefits.

"The first thing I do every morning, before I exercise and eat breakfast, is Transcendental Meditation. When I get home after a long day at the office, the first thing I do, before dinner, is Transcendental Meditation. The technique is extremely relaxing. It provides me with a practical, efficient, powerful respite from my very high level of activity. I absolutely count on it to keep me clear-headed, rested, and healthy."

—John Zamara, M.D., a specialist in cardiology and internal medicine, Orange County, California. Dr. Zamara has been practicing Transcendental Meditation for 21 years.

"I have long, complex days with many demands and many continuing pressures that spill over from day to day and week to week. I direct a clinical unit, take care of patients, teach medical students and residents, and carry out my research into neuroimaging. What I find is that Transcendental Meditation gives me a clearer mind, and I am able to focus my attention on areas that require the greatest amount of work. Stress doesn't accumulate; I return to each day with a freshness. Transcendental Meditation has enhanced my career and my life."

—Kelvin O. Lim, M.D., Assistant Professor of Psychiatry and Behavioral Sciences at Stanford University School of Medicine, Palo Alto, California. Dr. Lim has been practicing Transcendental Meditation for 13 years.

"Transcendental Meditation is like a daily vacation. It's a renewal for my body and calms my mind. I do a lot of writing and speaking, and it has given me a flood of creativity.

"I've always felt that Transcendental Meditation was an aid to my Christian growth. It never replaced my Christian growth, but it was an aid to it. In fact, I decided to commit my life to Christ after I'd been practicing Transcendental Meditation for 3 months.

"I would say to any Christian—to anyone of any religion—that Transcendental Meditation would benefit your life. It's a technique, a simple process that requires no belief. It is not a religion. There are so many thoughts that clutter the mind, and Transcendental Meditation is like taking a bath—it's very cleansing and very refreshing."

—Rev. Dr. Craig Overmyer, a pastoral counselor in Indianapolis, Indiana. Dr. Overmyer received his Master of Divinity in 1982 and his Doctorate of Ministry in 1985 from the Christian Theological Seminary in Indianapolis. He has been practicing Transcendental Meditation for 22 years.

"I wouldn't be able to fulfill my responsibilities as a rabbi to the level I expect of myself without Transcendental Meditation. I am better able to deal with the stresses of being with the sick and the dying, and the pressures of funerals, weddings, and bar mitzvahs because I have within me a considerable reservoir of calm. I am able to walk into a tense situation and naturally settle people down. They appreciate the ease and calm I bring to situations. But even more important, Transcendental Meditation has made me a better rabbi because it has given me an experience and insight into the profound depths of life. As a result, I am able to express a true depth of knowledge about my own tradition."

—Rabbi Alan Green of Beth Israel Synagogue in Winnipeg, Manitoba. Rabbi Green has been practicing Transcendental Meditation for 20 years.

"Transcendental Meditation is a tremendous stress buster. It's the most potent form of relaxation that I know of. After meditating just a few days, I noticed mental sharpness, less worry, and increased tolerance and ability to get along with people. It's one magnificent stroke that benefits my life in so many different ways."

—Glenn Pilling, actor, Los Angeles. Mr. Pilling has been practicing Transcendental Meditation for 14 months.

"I really appreciate the portability of Transcendental Meditation. I travel a lot, and I'm able to gain the benefits of meditating no matter what is happening around me. I recently was on a plane with very rambunctious children racing up and down the aisles. I just sat there enjoying my meditation. Afterwards, one of the parents came over and sat down next to me and said, 'What are you doing? You seem so peaceful!' Transcendental Meditation gives you equanimity. You can move through all kinds of situations during the day, coming from a place of peace, and then impart some of that peacefulness to others."

—Merrily Manthey, M.S., Director of the Institute for Executive Stress Management in Kent (greater Seattle area), Washington. She has been meditating for 22 years.

"I was out shopping recently with my husband— buying bikes for our kids at a mall. It was late, the mall was chaotic, and I was starting to get tired. On top of that, our son was coming home from college that night with three friends for dinner. Then I realized, I have nothing to worry about. I can go home and do my Transcendental Meditation, and I won't be tired anymore. I did—and I felt great, really refreshed afterward. I just wish I started when my friend first told me about it more than 20 years ago."

—Denise Droese, mother of four children, ages 4, 10, 12, and 20, Carmel, Indiana. Ms. Droese has been practicing Transcendental Meditation for one month.

CHAPTER 2

Unfolding
Full Mental Potential—
and Using it

I t's 8:30 a.m. and the phones are ringing off the
hook on the seventh floor of the World Financial
Center in Manhattan. *What do you think? What do you
think? What do you think? What do you think?*

"That's what I hear all day long," says Walter
Zimmermann, first Vice President at Lehmann Bros.
"Customers want to know what you think. There's a
lot at stake. If you're wrong, they can lose a lot of
money. And if you're right, they love you for it."

Mr. Zimmermann works in Lehmann's Global
Energy Department. For him each work day actually
starts the night before when he develops an "outlook"
for the next day. Where does he think any rally will
fail? Where does he think any decline will stop? Does
he think it will be an uptrend or a downtrend, or does
he expect a "congestion" day? On that basis he
decides: "How bullish am I? What's the best way of
taking advantage of that up move? Should I stay with
what I have? Should I add on? Should I reverse my
position?"

Mr. Zimmermann must develop an outlook for each hour, each day, each week, each month, and each quarter. Most of the people he deals with are short-term traders. They rarely hold anything for more than a week. They need to know from Mr. Zimmerman at each moment during the day, "Is this still your outlook? What do you think?"

Mr. Zimmermann has been practicing Transcendental Meditation for 23 years.

"My kind of work requires a unique combination of analytical skills and intuitive clarity. My tool is not the price charts or the news wires. My tool is the clarity of my awareness, with which I can pick up on things sooner than other people. I'm competing with some of the best minds out there. Everybody has the same information; everybody can look at the same price charts; everybody reads the same newspapers. But success comes to the person whose awareness can penetrate more deeply and, at the same time, be more sensitive to the onset of trend changes. If you haven't developed that kind of awareness, you're going to get crushed by the oil markets.

"Unfolding your mental potential is not simply time well spent; it's absolutely necessary if you're going to succeed. Transcendental Meditation gives me the clarity of mind and inner calm that does not get overshadowed or shaken by the high level of emotions and tension and anxiety that characterize this kind of work place."

Mr. Zimmermann started out with E.F. Hutton in Manhattan in 1984. The company was bought out by Shearson and has gone through several name changes to its current name, Lehmann Bros. Mr. Zimmermann has been highly successful through it all.

"This is a very stressful work environment. The petroleum market is the most volatile market out there, by a wide margin, and that volatility takes its toll. Normally you just don't last as long as I have. The people I started off with have burned out and gone on to other things. I attribute my endurance to Transcendental Meditation. Endurance has its advantages. If you endure, you remember things that other people weren't there to experience. You gather wisdom. If you've 'seen it all,' you basically know how to deal with it all.

"If someone asks me about Transcendental Meditation, I ask them, 'How valuable is mental clarity to you? How valuable are insight and innovation to you? How valuable is it for you to be able to see what other people don't see? If that's of value to you, then Transcendental Meditation is something you can do to get as much clarity and insight as you require.'"

Maharishi's Transcendental Meditation is not just a technique to reduce stress. It is much more than that. It is a practical, effective procedure for developing consciousness—for unfolding your full mental potential and using it in daily life.

Is There Time?

We have to be practical when it comes to time. Every day there are pressures, deadlines, and responsibilities to meet. There's a business deal to close, children to send off to school, a term paper to write. And tomorrow will probably be even busier.

So is it practical to take time to consider developing mental potential—much less do something about it—when there's so much to accomplish with so little time?

Perhaps intuitively we've always known that we weren't using our full potential in life, but due to the pressing demands on our time and energy today, we've had to put these considerations off until tomorrow— or to a distant future.

Is this being practical? Hardly.

If There's a Choice

Psychologists and psychiatrists estimate that we use between 5% and 10% of our mental potential. And there are days when even that figure may seem generous.

If you had a choice, wouldn't you prefer being able to draw upon more of your creativity and intelligence to resolve a problem at work, or organize your household, or take a test at school?

What could be more practical than having a clear, organized mind; or the ability to learn quickly and remember things accurately; or the capacity for broad comprehension along with the ability to focus sharply, for long periods of time?

Nothing could be more practical, and therefore nothing is more important than developing full mental potential—and using it.

How do you unfold mental potential through Transcendental Meditation?

Quite naturally. You simply gain access to the unlimited reservoir of energy, creativity, and intelligence that is located at the most settled, silent, fully awake level of your mind—the source of thought.

To understand how this is possible and to see how simple and natural it is, first we'll start with a few common experiences in daily life.

Excited Mind/Settled Mind

Two business professionals are reviewing the draft of a transaction over lunch at a crowded restaurant.

A high school student is working on a calculus problem with the television on.

Neither the business professionals nor the student are finding much success. Why? There is too much noise. Where there is more noise, there is more confusion.

Where there is more silence, there is more order, more intelligence.

So the business professionals meet later in a quiet conference room to complete the details of the transaction, and the student goes to his room to study.

Whenever we have something important to do, like study for a class or work out a business deal, or whenever we have something important to say, like a heart-to-heart talk with a family member or a close friend, we try to find a quiet place. Because when the mind is allowed to settle down, it naturally gains in clarity, comprehension, and decisiveness.

The Purpose of Transcendental Meditation

What is the purpose of Transcendental Meditation? Just this: Because of the constant demands on your time and energy, it's not often that you can get away to a quiet place for a long period of time. And even if you're able to get away, then because of the build-up of stress and tension, it can take a long while before your mind really begins to settle down.

What you need is a way to develop the ability for your mind to always remain clear and settled, a way to use the full potential of your mind at all times—even in the midst of the most hectic activity.

That's the purpose of Transcendental Meditation. It's a simple technique that allows the active mind to settle down—and continue settling down—until it reaches its own perfectly calm, collected state, where the body is deeply rested and the mind is silent, unbounded, and fully awake.

Transcendental Meditation is also very practical. It can be practiced anywhere at any time. Whether it's been an intense day at work or school, or a lazy Sunday, whether you're just home from an all-day downtown business meeting or a weekend boating trip, you can practice Transcendental Meditation and benefit from this settled state of awareness.

And exactly what is this most settled state?

It's the full potential of consciousness—a silent reservoir of unlimited creativity and intelligence found deep within your mind. And this reservoir, as we'll see later, is the same as the source of unlimited creativity and intelligence found deep within nature itself.

Dr. Christopher Hegarty is a management consultant, who speaks at more than 100 business conferences a year, on developing the fundamentals of competence. His client list includes chief executives at IBM, AT&T, Blue Cross, Xerox, and the United Airlines Pilots Association. He has been practicing Transcendental Meditation for over 20 years.

"The world is changing so fast, with so much new information to process, that to survive in business today—much less succeed—demands an optimal level of mental competence," says Dr. Hegarty.

"I consider Transcendental Meditation to be the single most effective technique available for developing this inner potential. Transcendental Meditation removes the stress and 'debris' from your mind and nervous system. It gives you access to your own deepest resources—what I have experienced to be a limitless source of energy and intelligence."

Thought Is the Basis of Activity

What is this reservoir of energy and intelligence that Dr. Hegarty and millions of other people experience twice a day during Transcendental Meditation? And where is it located?

Let's analyze it step by step, starting with thought.

Thought is the basis of activity: The design of a building begins with the thoughts of an architect; a legal brief begins with the thoughts of an attorney; a smooth-running household is based on the thoughts of a homemaker.

The clearer, more creative, more intelligent the thought, the more successful is the architectural design, the legal brief, the family's day.

What can make thought more intelligent and more powerful?

The way to make thought more powerful, according to Maharishi, is through contact with the reservoir of energy and intelligence deep within the mind, contact with the source of thought.

Thought: Energy and Intelligence

What is the source of thought? All day, every day we think innumerable thoughts. From the moment we wake up in the morning to the time we sleep at night, the mind is constantly thinking thoughts:

"Ten minutes to get the kids to school."

"I wonder who won the game last night?"

"Michael needs the computer file."

Is there anything common to these thoughts—and all the different thoughts that we think?

Yes—energy and intelligence.

• Energy—because all thoughts move; one thought follows another. This movement implies energy.

• Intelligence—because the energy takes a particular direction.

This means that all thoughts express some degree of energy and intelligence. And all day, every day, you are constantly thinking thoughts. That means you are constantly generating impulses of energy and intelligence.

What is the source of all this energy and intelligence? From where do thoughts arise?

While it is true that the stimulus for a particular thought may be a book or a conversation or a movie, the fact is, thoughts—impulses of energy and intelligence—arise from somewhere within us, from somewhere deep within the mind.

Where?

The Source of Thought

As we discussed earlier the mind can be

• Very noisy and excited

• Quiet and settled

• Perfectly settled and silent

As the mind settles down it naturally grows in creativity, intelligence, and energy. The deepest level of the mind is the field of maximum energy and intelligence.

It's here that we locate an unbounded reservoir of pure energy and creative intelligence. It is from here that all thoughts arise. This is the source of thought.

The source of thought, Maharishi says, is the field of pure consciousness, a "self-referral" level of awareness where consciousness is open only to itself—awake to its own full potential. It is silent, yet ready to function with maximum dynamism, clarity, and orderliness.

Transcendental Meditation is a simple, natural procedure—requiring neither concentration nor control—for refining mental activity and directly experiencing the source of thought.

Transcendental Meditation and Science

What does science tell us about this experience? From research in physiology and biochemistry, we learn that Transcendental Meditation reduces stress and anxiety and promotes a longer, healthier life. From psychology we learn that intelligence grows, memory improves, and learning ability increases.

And from the integration of modern physics and Transcendental Meditation, we learn something else: We learn of the deep connection between human beings and nature.

We learn that the source of intelligence within

each of us is the same as the source of the intelligence within nature, and that we have access to the unlimited creativity and intelligence of nature within our own consciousness. We learn what it means to unfold full mental potential—and use it.

To understand this connection between ourselves and nature, we first need a little background in physics.

Modern Physics Discovers the Unified Field— And What It Means to You

Physics investigates nature. We are a part of nature. So what can physics tell us about nature that can help us understand our own potential?

To consider this, first we'll review recent developments in physics and then relate them to ourselves.

Observe nature—a maple tree, a galaxy of stars, or an atom—and you observe the display of nature's intelligence. Everywhere in nature there is perfect orderliness, unfathomable energy, unlimited creativity, and infinite organizing power.

What is its source? Physics tells us that nature is structured in layers, that within the molecules are atoms, and that within atoms are subatomic particles. The deeper the layer, the greater the energy and organizing power.

The quest of science has always been to uncover deeper levels of nature's functioning and ultimately to discover the common source of the tree, the galaxy, the atom—the very source of the universe.

The Four Fundamental Forces of Nature

Forty years ago the basis of the universe was seen to be the four fundamental forces in nature and the so-called "matter fields." (The four forces are electromagnetism, which accounts for such things as electricity and chemical reactions; the weak force, which is responsible for such phenomena as radioactive decay; the strong force, which holds the nucleus of an atom together; and gravity, which keeps objects earthbound and planets in orbit.)

These force and matter fields constituted everything in the universe. Recently, physicists have uncovered even more powerful, more unified levels of nature. For example, at the level of "electro-weak unification," the electromagnetic force and the weak force become one. (See page 38.)

Discovery of the Source: the Unified Field

Now, the source of all the force and matter fields in the universe has been glimpsed by modern science in the supersymmetric unified quantum field theories of physics. It is called the unified field of natural law. It is a field of pure energy and intelligence, which underlies everything in creation and which is responsible for all forms and phenomena in the universe.

According to physics the entire universe emerges from the "self-interacting dynamics" of the unified field. And it is the unified field that gives rise to all the laws of nature that govern the entire universe.

Difficult to picture? Here's an analogy: The unified

field is like the sap within a tree. The sap, while color-less and formless itself, is nonetheless the source of the fragrant, red flower; the shiny, green leaf; the leathery, brown stem. The sap permeates the entire tree, manifesting itself as flower, leaf, and stem. In the same way, the unified field underlies and pervades the universe. It is the basis of the infinite energy, cre-ativity, and intelligence displayed in nature. It is the basis of everything in the universe, including our-selves. Now, what does that mean to you?

Displaying the Unlimited Creativity and Intelligence of Nature in Your Life

The unified field deep within nature is a field of unlimited energy, creativity, and intelligence. The source of thought deep within every individual is also a field of unlimited energy, creativity, and intelligence.

Is there a connection between them? Yes.

Maharishi states: "Modern physics has recently glimpsed the unified field of all the laws of nature. Since ancient times the unified field has been described by Vedic science—a complete science of conscious-ness—as the field of pure consciousness, the field of infinite energy, creativity, and intelligence underlying man and nature. Through Transcendental Medita-tion, pure consciousness—the unified field—can be enlivened at the source of thought deep within the mind of every human being.

"This means that we can display the infinite creativity, intelligence, and dynamism of nature in our own life. This is our natural birthright."

33

John S. Hagelin, Ph.D., a member of an elite group of scientists who are at the forefront of research in unified field theories, agrees.

Dr. Hagelin is an expert on supersymmetric unified quantum field theories and has published over 90 papers on the subject in leading physics journals. Dr. Hagelin received his doctorate in physics from Harvard and has conducted research at two of the top laboratories in the world for advanced particle physics—the European Laboratory for Particle Physics (CERN) in Geneva, Switzerland, and the Stanford Linear Accelerator Center (SLAC) in Palo Alto, California.

Since 1976 Dr. Hagelin has studied Maharishi's descriptions of pure consciousness in the light of modern physics. Recent advances in quantum physics, Dr. Hagelin says, provide "substantial evidence that the unified field and pure consciousness are not two separate fields, but one and the same."

As Chairman of the Department of Physics and Director of the Institute of Science, Technology and Public Policy at Maharishi International University in Fairfield, Iowa, Dr. Hagelin is a recognized world authority on unified field theories and a pre-eminent scholar in the dynamics of human consciousness.

"It is clear that the unified field is ultimately the origin of all attributes in the universe," Dr. Hagelin says. "Any property of existence—electric charge or color charge—must have its dynamical origin in the structure of the unified field itself.

"The properties of intelligence, dynamism, and self-interaction can also be located in the structure of the unified field, suggesting a link between the unified field and the 'ground state,' or most fundamental state, of consciousness.

"When one examines the properties of the unified field in detail, one discovers all the properties of pure consciousness."

What Does All of This Mean?

It means that the full potential of your mind is the same as the total potential of nature's intelligence. It means that you have the innate capacity to use and display the unlimited energy, creativity, and intelligence of nature in your own life.

And for this you only need to restore the natural connection—through Transcendental Meditation—between the thinking mind and the source of thought, between the active mind and the unified field. When you make this connection, you grow in creativity and intelligence, reduce stress and fatigue, and enjoy greater happiness and more progress and accomplishments in your life. You gain the support of nature for everything you do.

"Being able to go to that silent place within me everyday has unlocked an incredible storehouse of creative potential," says Chris Boas, a third-year law student at the University of San Francisco Law School. "Since I've been meditating, good ideas just seem to come easily. I feel that there's no end to what I can accomplish."

Chris is studying intellectual property and technology licensing—"high technology law." He's been meditating for 12 years.

"The ability to think clearly is the main requirement in law school. The knowledge in law school is really not that difficult. There's a lot of it, but the underlying concepts are really not that complicated. What's difficult is thinking clearly under pressure. People who do well in law school are those who handle that pressure, especially during final exam time.

"Since I've been meditating, my mind stays relaxed and alert, and I can think through things clearly and logically, even under pressure. I can retain information more easily, and I can access it more quickly whenever I need it.

"I also have a deeper keel in life. The waves that come at me are the same, the pressures that come at me are the same, but it's so much easier to keep my equilibrium. I wasn't like that before I started meditating. It was easy for me to get flustered when there was a lot of pressure. It would snowball into a cycle where it was very hard to get back on track. I find that meditating twice a day helps me stay on track day after day after day."

To a student entering law school, Chris says, "Transcendental Meditation makes education enjoyable. Many people find the first year of law school to be a painful experience or, at least, a chaotic one.

Transcendental Meditation allows you to enjoy the process. And instead of feeling like you have to compete with everybody else, you'll feel like you have a lot to give to everybody else."

Experiencing Self-Referral Awareness through Transcendental Meditation

Maharishi comments: "In Transcendental Meditation the conscious mind comes to a state of self-referral awareness, which is the simplest form of human awareness where consciousness is open only to itself. This self-referral state of consciousness is the unified field of natural law.

"The supersymmetric unified field theories of physics have glimpsed this state of unity, which, through its own self-interacting dynamics, expresses itself as diversified forms and phenomena in creation.

"When the conscious mind identifies itself with the unified field through the process of Transcendental Meditation, then human awareness is open to its full potential, which is the total potential of nature's intelligence.

"As a result, thinking and action spontaneously become more and more in accord with the evolutionary power of natural law. By enlivening this most basic level, Transcendental Meditation is that one simple procedure which can raise the life of every individual to its full dignity in which perfect health, happiness, and success are the natural features of daily life."

THEORY

Discovery of the Unified Field
as the Source of
All the Laws of Nature

QUANTUM PHYSICS

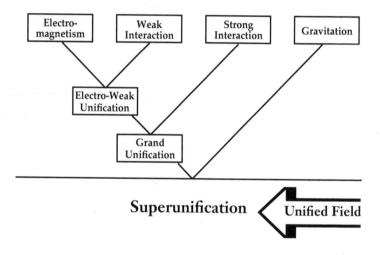

Progress in theoretical physics during the past two decades has led to a progressively more unified understanding of the fundamental forces of nature. This has culminated in the recent discovery of completely unified field theories.

PRACTICE

Experience of the Unified Field
in Human Awareness
through:

TRANSCENDENTAL MEDITATION

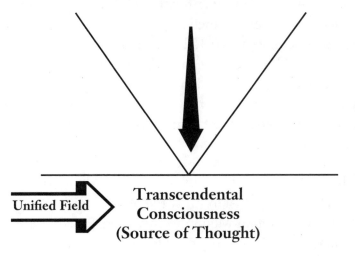

Unified Field

**Transcendental
Consciousness
(Source of Thought)**

Transcendental Meditation allows the active thinking mind to settle down to transcendental consciousness, the field of pure intelligence, where the mind is silent, unbounded, and fully awake within itself. This self-referral state of consciousness is the unified field of natural law.

The Mind-Body Connection:
Science Studies Transcendental Meditation

When scientists first decided to study the effects of Transcendental Meditation, they looked to the body.

Why? Because there is an intimate connection between the mind and the body. Researchers knew that for every state of consciousness there is a corresponding style of functioning of the physiology. For example, when you sleep at night your brain waves slow down, as do your heart rate, breath rate, and other physiological functions.

So scientists predicted that if the mind does, in fact, quiet down and become more expanded, more awake during Transcendental Meditation, then due to the close coordination between mind and body, the entire physiology must change as well—and it must be measurable.

The First Research on Transcendental Meditation

The first scientist to study the physiological effects of Transcendental Meditation was Dr. Robert Keith Wallace at UCLA in 1968. Dr. Wallace found that during Transcendental Meditation, the entire system gained a unique and profound state of rest and relaxation—far deeper than ordinary eyes-closed rest. He also observed biochemical changes indicative of reduced stress, and changes in EEG, or brain wave patterns, that indicated a state of "heightened inner wakefulness" or restful alertness.

The State of Restful Alertness:
A Fourth Major State of Consciousness

Analyzing his findings and comparing them to research on the three major states of consciousness, Dr. Wallace arrived at a remarkable conclusion. Transcendental Meditation produced a fourth major state of consciousness—a unique state of "restful alertness"—different from waking, dreaming, and sleeping states of consciousness, but also essential to the health and well-being of an individual.

Dr. Wallace's findings were published in the March 1970 issue of *Science*.

Since that initial study there have been more than 500 scientific studies on Transcendental Meditation, conducted at 210 independent universities and research institutions in 33 countries, including Harvard Medical School, University of Chicago, Stanford, and UCLA.

Much of the research has been published in leading scientific journals, including *The American Journal of Physiology, International Journal of Neuroscience, Psychosomatic Medicine, American Psychologist,* and the *Journal of Conflict Resolution.*

The research has documented the effects of the Transcendental Meditation program in every area of life, including mind, body, behavior, and society.

Brain Wave Coherence

One of the most significant findings shows that Transcendental Meditation produces a unique ordering, or coherence, in brain wave patterns among the different parts of the brain. And the longer a person practices Transcendental Meditation, the higher the EEG coherence.

Dr. Wallace, who now is Chairman of the Physiology Department at Maharishi International University and one of the world's leading experts on the research on Transcendental Meditation, explains the meaning of this finding:

"Higher EEG coherence produced during Transcendental Meditation indicates that the technique 'optimizes brain functioning.' This means that the brain functions in a more coherent, integrated style during Transcendental Meditation than during the usual waking, dreaming, and sleeping states of consciousness.

"Many psychological studies have shown that the higher EEG coherence gained during Transcendental Meditation is associated with increased intelligence and creativity and higher moral reasoning."

What is the cause of EEG coherence? "The increased orderliness and integration between the different parts of the brain corresponds to the direct experience of the self-referral state of pure consciousness—the unified field—gained during Transcendental Meditation," Dr. Wallace says.

Unfolding Full Mental Potential

What does "optimizing brain functioning" mean in daily life? It means unfolding the full creative potential of the mind—and using it. And using this full potential means enjoying the state of enlightenment in every aspect of daily life.

"Every day I experience a higher level of mental 'peak performance' from Transcendental Meditation than I experienced by chance during those 7 games of the World Series," says Buddy Biancalana, former shortstop for the Kansas City Royals and a star of the 1985 World Series.

Sportswriters called the World Series one of the most exciting in recent memory, and it turned Buddy Biancalana into a national hero. Kansas City faced off against the St. Louis Cardinals. The Royals fell behind three games to one and then stormed back to win it in seven games. Buddy's sparkling, acrobatic defense and unexpected clutch hitting helped propel Kansas City to the world championship. It was the best 7 games of baseball in Buddy's professional career, and it came when hundreds of millions of people all over the world were watching on television.

"I was deep in the 'zone' during the whole World Series," Buddy recalls. "I had a tremendously deep level of focus, to the point where I felt I couldn't do anything wrong. I felt like every play was going to go my way—and it did. It was a level of clarity I had never experienced playing baseball prior to that time—or in any other aspect of my life—and I never reached it again until I learned Transcendental Meditation."

Today, Buddy is a players' agent, scouting and signing professional baseball players and negotiating their contracts. He has been meditating for 8 months.

"Now, when I get up in the morning, I know it's going to be a great day. There may be obstacles, I may have things to work out in my business, but the core of me is always feeling fabulous, no matter what is going on around me. Every day is a great day."

The following research charts represent a few of the many studies conducted on the effects of Transcendental Meditation for developing mental potential. The charts represent the average benefits of the group studied.

Greater Orderliness
of Brain Functioning

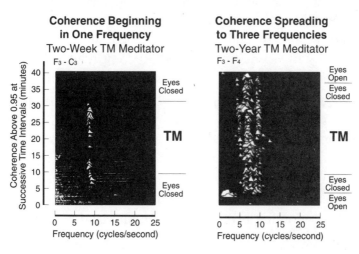

**Coherence Beginning
in One Frequency**
Two-Week TM Meditator

**Coherence Spreading
to Three Frequencies**
Two-Year TM Meditator

EEG coherence increases between and within the cerebral hemispheres during Transcendental Meditation. EEG coherence is a quantitative index of the degree of long-range spatial ordering of the brain waves. The chart on the left shows that for a 2-week meditator, EEG coherence increased during the period of meditation. The chart on the right, of a 2-year meditator, shows high levels of coherence even before meditation began, spreading of coherence to high and lower frequencies about half way through the meditation period, and continuing high coherence even into the eyes-opened period after meditation.

Reference I: The Coherence Spectral Array (COSPAR) and its application to the study of spatial ordering in the EEG, *Proceedings of the San Diego Biomedical Symposium* 15: 1976. **Reference II:** Electrophysiologic characteristics of respiratory suspension periods occurring during the practice of the Transcendental Meditation program, *Psychosomatic Medicine* 46: 267-276, 1984.

"**For me the experience of settled inner wakefulness** and expanded awareness during Transcendental Meditation is the real foundation for successful decision-making. After meditating I have the mental clarity and alertness for laser-like focus on the details and, at the same time, for broad comprehension so I don't get lost in the details. I find myself continuously growing in insight and intuition, as well as in the ability to focus and analyze. In my experience, if you can have those qualities together at the same time, you're going to make the right decisions—not only for your own success, but for the progress and well-being of others. Over my years in business, Transcendental Meditation has been a real competitive advantage."

—Steve Rubin, Chairman and CEO, United Fuels International, Inc., one of the world's largest international energy brokerage firms.

Broader Comprehension and Improved Ability to Focus

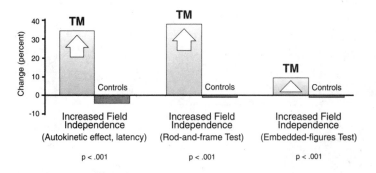

Field independence has been associated with a greater ability to assimilate and structure experience, greater organization of mind and cognitive clarity, improved memory, greater creative expression, and a stable internal frame of reference. The results show that practice of the Transcendental Meditation technique develops greater field independence. This improvement in Transcendental Meditation meditators is remarkable because it was previously thought that these basic perceptual abilities do not improve beyond early adulthood.

Reference I: Influence of Transcendental Meditation upon autokinetic perception, *Perceptual Motor Skills* 39: 1031-1034, 1974.
Reference II: Longitudinal effects of the Transcendental Meditation and TM-Sidhi program on cognitive ability and cognitive style, *Perceptual and Motor Skills* 62: 731–738, 1986.

Increased Creativity

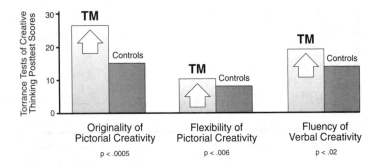

This study used the Torrance Tests of Creative Thinking to measure figural and verbal creativity in a control group and in a group that subsequently learned the Transcendental Meditation technique. On the posttest 5 months later, the Transcendental Meditation group scored significantly higher on figural originality and flexibility and on verbal fluency.

Reference I: The TM technique and creativity: A longitudinal study of Cornell University undergraduates, *Journal of Creative Behavior* 13: 169-190, 1979. **Reference II:** A psychological investigation into the source of the effect of the Transcendental Meditation technique, (Ph.D. dissertation, York University) *Dissertations Abstracts International* 38, 7-B: 3372–3373, 1978.

Improved Perception and Memory

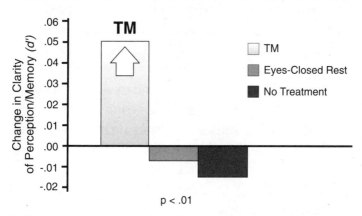

p < .01

College students instructed in Transcendental Meditation displayed significant improvements in performance over a 2-week period on a perceptual and short-term memory test involving the identification of familiar letter sequences presented rapidly. They were compared with subjects randomly assigned to a routine of twice-daily rest with eyes closed, and with subjects who made no change in their daily routine.

Meditation and flexibility of visual perception and verbal problem solving, *Memory and Cognition* 10: 207–215, 1982.

"The most powerful benefit that I've experienced from Transcendental Meditation is that it makes my mind much sharper. It allows the haziness in my mind to be cleared away so that everything makes sense to me and connects to my own ideas. From that level it's much easier to study, and every subject that I study has a much more penetrating effect. I can't imagine being a student without it. I've also found that once I have that clarity, all good things in life are drawn to me. When I'm feeling clear and the stress is gone, everything just naturally supports me and comes my way."

—Jennie Rothenberg is a 1993 National Merit Scholar and a first-year literature major at Maharishi International University in Fairfield, Iowa. (Maharishi International University integrates the arts, sciences, and professions with the study and development of consciousness through the practice of Transcendental Meditation. Maharishi International University is accredited to the Ph.D. level by the North Central Association of Colleges and Schools.)

Development of Intelligence

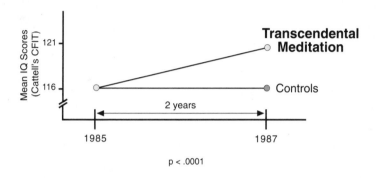

p < .0001

Students at Maharishi International University in Fairfield, Iowa, who regularly practiced Transcendental Meditation, increased significantly in intelligence over a 2-year period, compared to control subjects from another Iowa university. This finding corroborates the results of two other studies showing increased IQ in Maharishi International University students.

Reference I: Transcendental Meditation and improved performance on intelligence-related measures: A longitudinal study, *Personality and Individual Differences* 12: 1105-1116, 1991. **Reference II:** Longitudinal effects of the Transcendental Meditation and TM-Sidhi program on cognitive ability and cognitive style, *Perceptual and Motor Skills* 62: 731–738, 1986.

CHAPTER 3

Healthy Mind/
Healthy Body

"I believe that your mind controls your body, and I'm convinced that Transcendental Meditation has kept me not just mentally healthy, but also physically healthy and in very good shape," says Mike Fitzgerald, Director of the Washington State Department of Community Trade and Economic Development. "I have a lot to do, and I would never have the high energy level that I have without Transcendental Meditation."

Mr. Fitzgerald directs a newly formed department with a $700 million annual budget, 420 employees, and a broad and diverse range of responsibilities.

On a typical day Mr. Fitzgerald will help the governor and the state legislature formulate their policies on GATT and NAFTA. He'll make decisions on what kind of taxation package his department will put to the legislature to give incentives for small businesses. He'll meet with a group of community leaders to try to determine how to restructure a local economic development grant that will allow them to take new initiatives in their community. He'll also meet with local government representatives to determine how to improve and expand access to the state's early childhood education programs.

Mr. Fitzgerald learned Transcendental Meditation at a friend's recommendation.

"I notice, almost instantly after meditating, a relief from the pressures of the day, and a new clarity, a new freshness, and a new energy," says Mr. Fitzgerald, whose day starts at 5:30 a.m. and ends at 7:30 p.m. when he gets home to his family in Issaquah, a city 10 miles east of Seattle.

"I'm in very good physical shape, and Transcendental Meditation has helped me a lot with that because it keeps stress at a minimum. I don't overeat. Meditating also helps to keep me calm and thoughtful and restful and reflective. It's my lifeline in a very chaotic world."

Mr. Fitzgerald says Transcendental Meditation can play a key role in solving social ills.

"The tendency of our society is to deal with events and symptoms, not causes," he says. "We deal with the symptoms of too much violence, not the causes of it. We deal with the symptoms of disease, not the causes of it. The basic cause is that people are full of stress. Transcendental Meditation goes to the heart of the problem. It releases stress and makes individuals healthier and more self-reliant, and puts them in a position where they can start to solve their own problems."

"It is fortunate for the field of health today that one technique exists to take care of the very basis of an individual's life—pure consciousness—and thereby to restore and maintain perfect health on all levels of mind, body, and surroundings." —*Maharishi*

What Are the Trillion Dollars Used for?

The United States has one of the most technologically sophisticated and advanced health care systems in the world. Each year we spend over one trillion dollars on health care—more than 12% of the entire gross national product (GNP). By the year 2000 that amount could spiral to as much as 18%.

What are the trillion dollars used for? Preventing illness? Securing the health and well-being of every American?

No. As just about everyone knows, that huge sum of money is used mainly for treating disease. And according to many health experts, up to 90% of those diseases could have been prevented.

How? By effectively reducing stress, which is a prime causal factor in a majority of disorders—from headaches and the common cold to serious illnesses such as heart disease and many forms of cancer.

What Is Stress?

To understand how you can reduce stress and therefore prevent disease, first we should define it. Stress is not a deadline to meet at work, a term paper, or even a traffic tie-up during rush hour. Stress is how we react, physically and mentally, to these experiences.

Some days we're better at it; some days we're not. If we've slept well at night and wake up fresh and rested, we're apt to handle any demand during the day far better than if we run into it, headlong, on a Friday afternoon at the end of a long week.

Stress, then, can be understood to be any structural or material abnormality in the body (tight neck muscles, high blood pressure, tension headaches, etc.) that is caused by overloading the machinery of experience, the senses.

Any overload can cause it. The sudden flash of a bulb from a camera can create stress in the eyes. Too much exertion or excitement can cause stress—or not enough rest. Any experience, positive or negative, can create stress if the system is unable to handle it.

Is Stress the Spice of Life?

Some say that stress is the spice of life. People who thrive on the continual stimulation of new challenges, new responsibilities, new pressures would hate to live without stress.

It's true that new opportunities and new challenges are essential for a fulfilling life. Eliminating stress from your life does not mean eliminating these challenges. Rather, it means eliminating their negative side-effects—chronic fatigue, anxiety, headaches, indigestion, insomnia, etc.—which severely restrict your capacity to be healthy, successful, and enjoy what you do.

How to Manage Stress?

How, then, can you live your life fully and not be victimized by stress?

There are many "stress management techniques" available today that try to minimize stress by training people how to better organize their time, their responsibilities, and their work and home environments.

These techniques often give advice on how to avoid high-pressure situations, recommend mental imagery exercises, and advocate changes in lifestyle to reduce stress. Some suggest de-escalating career goals.

Are these the basics of stress management?

No. They may be helpful in their own right, but they are not the "bottom line" on stress management.

What is the bottom line?

Rest. The very deep rest gained during 20 minutes of Maharishi's Transcendental Meditation allows the body to rejuvenate itself and throw off the accumulated stress and fatigue that has built up over years. It helps to normalize high blood pressure, reduce high cholesterol levels, improve bronchial asthma, provide relief from insomnia—even improve reaction time and athletic performance.

Without this rest, you can only hope to "manage" stress and struggle to organize your schedule to cope with growing stress in life, not eliminate it.

Don't Manage Stress, Prevent and Eliminate It

With this rest you don't just manage stress, you prevent new stress from accumulating today and you eliminate stress built up from the past. Research shows that you'll improve your health, increase your energy, and promote the clarity of your mind and the creativity and orderliness of your thinking. Then you'll be better prepared to meet all of the responsibilities in your life without creating more stress and strain and without reducing or shying away from any new commitment or challenge. At the same time you'll grow in the capacity to enjoy life to its fullest.

"I have been using Transcendental Meditation in my practice as a stress-reduction modality for the past 20 years," says Steele Belok, M.D., clinical instructor of medicine at Harvard Medical School. "I have found that it is not only an effective tool to use in anxiety-related disorders, but it also has significant physiological effects. I have seen positive effects on hypertension, cholesterol, asthma, and insomnia. In addition, for patients who are healthy and who are interested in prevention and health promotion, I have found Transcendental Meditation to be highly effective in enhancing their physical and mental well-being. These effects have been corroborated by a growing body of scientific literature showing the effectiveness of Transcendental Meditation in these and other areas."

Reducing the Effects of Traumatic Stress

There are the normal stresses and strains of daily life—and then there is the devastating impact of *traumatic stress*. Transcendental Meditation has also been found to be a potent antidote to the effects of extreme stress—what doctors have termed "post-traumatic stress syndrome." For example, a 3-month study of Vietnam veterans found that veterans who learned Transcendental Meditation improved significantly compared to veterans who were participating in a counseling program. The veterans practicing Transcendental Meditation were found to be less emotionally numb and had reduced alcohol abuse, insomnia, depression, and anxiety. They also showed a decreased severity of "delayed stress syndrome" (*Journal of Counseling and Development* 64: 212-214, 1985).

Transcendental Meditation also helps those who are recovering from the trauma of a serious illness, and those who have suffered through the stress of other major traumas, such as a serious auto accident.

Martha Gray, 48, is a data architect who develops computing systems for the Boeing Company in Seattle. In March 1992 Martha was diagnosed as having breast cancer. She had surgery—a lumpectomy—and afterwards underwent six months of chemotherapy and then radiation treatments. Doctors told Martha that her prognosis was good. But by the end of her treatments, Martha was in a deep depression.

"I went to a breast cancer support group, and I discovered that depression was almost an accepted way of life," Martha recalls. "The majority of the women—and I mean the *majority* of the women—who were in that group were on some sort of anti-depressants. After all that I had been through, I realized that I just did not want to live my life in anxiety and fear."

Martha had been doing a lot of reading and had heard about Transcendental Meditation. She learned the technique at the Transcendental Meditation Center in Seattle on June 19, 1993.

"It has absolutely changed everything for me," Martha says. "My outlook is completely different. I'm positive; I'm happy. Transcendental Meditation releases the stress. That's been the key. Before I would try to laugh off the anxiety, or disregard it, or stuff it back down, or try to ignore it, or try to be brave—all the things you try to do to manipulate the fear and try to keep going. With Transcendental Meditation the stress is released and it's gone. It's been tremendously freeing.

"When people talk about all the problems that a cancer patient faces, they forget to realize that the family and spouse also go through a tremendous amount of anxiety and anguish and fear. Because my husband, Fred, started Transcendental Meditation also, it's been a wonderful thing for him, too."

Fred Gray, 48, is a final-assembly flight-line inspector for Boeing. He gives each Boeing 747 a final review before the $160 million aircraft is delivered to an airline. Fred says that Transcendental Meditation keeps him relaxed on the job—"I have a very stressful occupation"—and happier within himself. He also sees a big change in Martha and in their relationship together.

"Transcendental Meditation has calmed Martha a great deal," Fred says. "She doesn't dwell on the fear of the possible recurrence of her illness. Her health has skyrocketed. Chemotherapy had really disrupted her body. Now she's vivacious and healthy and alert. Since we started meditating, we also have a much better relationship. We look at each other and nod in agreement. We don't have to express so many things verbally anymore; we just understand what's going on."

Martha encourages others facing recovery from a major illness to practice the technique.

"Transcendental Meditation is the key to regaining a sense of well-being and purpose in your life. After having what some people would consider a catastrophic illness, it's a must. It's something that restores a sense of balance and enthusiasm for life. You won't be afraid, and you'll be able to make plans for the future without some dread. I honestly wish I would have discovered this a long time ago, because in my own mind, my life would have been different."

Martha has just had a 2-year check-up and her doctors say that everything is fine.

"It helps so much to be able to sit down twice a day and just quiet ourselves," Martha says. "Transcendental Meditation has created a stress-free, happy way of life for both of us."

"I had so much physical and emotional stress from the accident," says Gail Tomura, an artist living in West Los Angeles. "Transcendental Meditation is the first thing that helped because it gives me such profound rest. It's finally allowing that deep stress to be released. In the 3 months I've been meditating, I've made more progress with all of my treatments than I have in the past 8 years."

Gail was a bright 28-year-old graduate student working towards a masters' degree in fine arts at Claremont College in southern California. On July 18, 1986, she was driving at dusk along a narrow winding road near Fullerton when she was hit head-on by car speeding at 60 miles an hour.

Gail was lucky to be alive. She broke a leg, an arm, and two ribs, fractured her skull, and suffered what her doctors called a "mild-to-moderate" head injury. She began an intensive program of physical therapy and cognitive therapy. She said that she felt like she was walking with a thick fog around her head. She had to relearn to read, concentrate, follow directions, and find things on a map. She had been an avid reader, devouring three to four books a month. Now, if she was lucky, she could read three to four books in a year.

Determined to recover, she made slow but steady progress for 6 years. She wasn't back to 100% yet, but she was getting close, when on June 24, 1992, Gail was in another car accident. It was minor—no broken bones—but it somehow brought back her old symptoms. Her headaches returned and so did her backaches and neckaches. Gail's doctor put her on an intensive program of 4-days-a-week physical therapy and recommended counseling. It didn't help. She tried some alternative therapies. She didn't get any better. She said that she lost hope and began to sink into a depression.

Gail had read something about Transcendental Meditation and decided to give it a try. On December 4, 1993, she learned the technique at the Transcendental Meditation Center in Pacific Palisades.

"The fog is gone," Gail says now. "My mind is clearer than it has been since the accident. I am able to read more, and my comprehension is excellent.

"Before I started meditating I used to have tremendous fatigue doing anything. If I had one day of activity, I had to have a full day of rest in bed. If I cooked a meal or went to the grocery store, I was exhausted. Now, for the first time in 8 years, I don't have a fatigue problem. I have much more energy, and I rarely get tired. I feel healthier—mentally, emotionally, physically—than I have since my accident."

Gail's art career is taking off. She does painting and drawing, and for the first time she is finding that she doesn't have to solicit shows; curators are starting to call her, and collectors are buying more of her work.

"Transcendental Meditation has helped me in so many ways. It has given me hope of being able to get beyond anything in my life—beyond chronic pain, beyond my own insecurities, beyond anything."

Transcendental Meditation over Time—
Slowing Down the Aging Process

We know that stress—normal daily stress and severe traumatic stress—is at the basis of almost all diseases and disorders. We also know that stress greatly accelerates the aging process. Nearly 15 years ago, researchers began to study the effects of Transcendental Meditation on aging. Not surprisingly, considering the role of stress in aging, researchers found that long-term practice of Transcendental Meditation can promote a significantly younger biological age.

Chronological Age/Biological Age

To understand how this could happen, first it helps to understand a little about the aging process.

People age at different rates. According to most theories, the causes of aging are complex. They include heredity, the stress of daily living, and prior illnesses. But it all adds up to wear and tear on the system. For example, Charles is 48 years old according to his birth certificate, but his doctor knows otherwise. His doctor knows that because of intense job stress, Charles has the physiology of an average 60-year-old. The doctor recommends that Charles cut back on his workload and stop smoking, and he prescribes special medication for his high blood pressure.

Paul, on the other hand, is 49 years old and in good shape. Paul's doctor says that he has the physiology of a man 5 years younger. He gets a clean bill of health.

There is a difference between chronological age

and biological age. Chronological age is fixed; it's your age based on your birth certificate—the number of years you have lived. Biological age isn't fixed; it is an indication of your overall state of health compared to the norm in the general population. Scientists can use several tests, such as measurements of systolic blood pressure, auditory threshold, and near-point vision, to distinguish an individual's biological age from his actual chronological age.

Research on Transcendental Meditation and Aging

The first scientist to study the effects of Transcendental Meditation on aging was Dr. Robert Keith Wallace, the same physiologist who pioneered Transcendental Meditation research as a graduate student at UCLA in 1968. Twelve years after his first Transcendental Meditation study was published in *Science*, Dr. Wallace published his research on Transcendental Meditation and aging in the *International Journal of Neuroscience* (16: 53–58, 1982).

12 Years Younger

Dr. Wallace found that subjects with an average chronological age of 50 years, who had been practicing Transcendental Meditation for over 5 years, had a biological age 12 years younger than their chronological age. That means a 55-year-old meditator had the physiology of a 43-year-old.

Several of the subjects in the study were found to have a biological age 27 years younger than their chronological age. This study has since been replicated several times. Other studies have also shown the beneficial effects of Transcendental Meditation on the aging process.

• A higher level of plasma dehydroepiandrosterone sulfate (DHEAS) is a hormonal marker of younger biological age. A study found DHEAS to be significantly higher for 326 adult Transcendental Meditation technique practitioners than for 972 age- and sex-matched controls. These differences were largest for the oldest age categories. (*Journal of Behavioral Medicine,* 15(4): 327-341, 1992.)

• A study randomly assigned residents of 8 homes for the elderly (average age 81 years) to one of the following programs: Transcendental Meditation; an active thinking (mindfulness) program; a relaxation program; or a control group with no treatment. The Transcendental Meditation group improved most on a wide range of physical and mental health measures. In addition to reporting that they felt younger, the Transcendental Meditation group actually lived longer. After 3 years, all members were still living, in contrast to lower survival rates for the other experimental groups, and a 63% survival rate for the 478 other residents who did not participate in the study. (*Journal of Personality and Social Psychology,* 57(6): 950-964, 1989.)

Are these findings surprising? "No, not when you consider that all the major factors associated with longevity, such as hypertension and cholesterol, have been shown to improve with the regular practice of the Transcendental Meditation technique," Dr. Wallace says.

"Transcendental Meditation has been shown to significantly improve cardiovascular health, work satisfaction, positive health habits, physical function, happiness rating, self-health rating, intelligence, and mental health. The result is a younger biological age."

"**I'm never tired since I started meditating,**" says Ann Hurley, 75. "I've got a lot of energy. I work at my son's law office, and I run circles around the two women in the office. It's two stories, and I run up and down the stairs all day. One of the women said to me, 'Don't you ever get tired?' I stopped and thought, and I realized that this hasn't happened to me since Transcendental Meditation. I'm not tired anymore."

Ann worked for DuPont for 33 years before taking an early retirement in 1983. Then, in 1987, she went to work for her son in Wilmington, Delaware. She started by filling in as a temporary receptionist over the lunch hour, and now she works from nine o'clock in the morning until five or six o'clock at night, doing filing, legal work, and accounting. She brings extra work home and does accounting on her computer. She started meditating in 1988.

"Transcendental Meditation has made my mind clearer. Now I've got this desire to study; I want to know more. Before I just goofed off like everybody else. Now people ask me, 'Why do you read all the time?' I say, 'Transcendental Meditation has woken up my mind. I want to know more about everything.'

"I'm enjoying life, really enjoying life. That's what

I do now. I go to work and I go on trips and I look forward to the next day and how beautiful it's going to be, which I never did before. Transcendental Meditation has changed my whole outlook on life—that life is really worth living."

An Effective Solution to Spiraling Health Costs

What are the combined benefits of reduced stress, better health, and a younger biological age? Among the many advantages is a dramatic reduction in health care use—and with it, an effective answer to the crisis of spiraling health care costs.

A 5-year nationwide study of more than 2,000 Transcendental Meditation practitioners found that the Transcendental Meditation group made 55% fewer health insurance claims than did the population norms. The group had less than half of the hospital admissions and outpatient visits of other professional groups. They also had lower sickness rates in all categories, including 87% less hospitalization for heart disease and 55% less for cancer. In addition, people practicing Transcendental Meditation who were over 40 years of age had an even higher percentage reduction in insurance utilization compared to the norm for their age group (*Psychosomatic Medicine* 4: 493-507, 1987).

On the basis of this insurance study, and hundreds of other findings on the technique, physicians and other health care professionals now see Transcendental Meditation as a practical, cost-effective solution to the health care crisis.

"We are trying to solve the health care crisis by rearranging who pays for the sickness," says Hari Sharma, M.D., F.R.C.P.C. "What we need to do is keep people from falling sick in the first place. That is true health care reform; then we'll save money in the best possible way by keeping people healthy."

Dr. Sharma is Professor of Pathology and Director of Cancer Prevention and Natural Products Research at The Ohio State University College of Medicine. He is a consultant to the National Institutes of Health, Alternative Medicine Section, and has lectured on preventive medicine to medical audiences around the world, including the World Health Organization.

"In truth, the health care crisis is a crisis of stress. There's an epidemic of stress, both in individuals and in society as a whole. Stress breaks down physical and mental health in the individual and creates biochemicals that are destructive to the physical body.

"In multiple published research studies, Transcendental Meditation has been shown to be the most effective technique for reducing stress and rebalancing the biochemicals in the body to produce improved physical and mental health. This has been corroborated by research showing that Transcendental Meditation reduces health care utilization by 50%."

Dr. Sharma is the author of *Freedom from Disease— How to Control Free Radicals, a Major Cause of Aging and Disease.* He practices Transcendental Meditation and says that the technique should be widely applied as part of reforming America's health care system.

"Transcendental Meditation is a major preventive technology. Like everything else in prevention, Transcendental Meditation should be covered by health care providers. That way we can prevent forthcoming disorders that are extremely costly—not only financially, but also in terms of human pain and suffering. Transcendental Meditation would help the individual, society, and the federal government. It would help everyone."

The following charts represent just a few of the numerous research studies conducted on the physiological effects of Transcendental Meditation, and their benefits to health.

Natural Change in Breathing

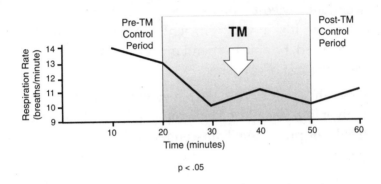

p < .05

Subjects were measured for changes in breathing rate during the practice of the Transcendental Meditation technique. Breath rate fell from about 14 breaths per minute to about 11 breaths per minute, indicating the Transcendental Meditation technique produces a state of rest and relaxation. The change in breath rate is natural, effortless, and comfortable.

A wakeful hypometabolic physiologic state, *American Journal of Physiology* 22: 795–799, 1971.

"I used to get real stressed in college. I knew that medical school would be even more stressful. Transcendental Meditation has been perfect for me. It's so relaxing. It's a very efficient way for me to get re-charged, be able to spend more time studying, and get more out of my day."

—Sarah Church, first-year medical student, Emory University School of Medicine, Atlanta. Ms. Church has been practicing Transcendental Meditation for 6 months.

Physiological Indicators
of Deep Rest

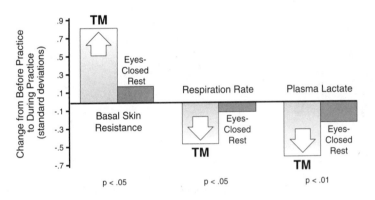

A meta-analysis, the preferred scientific procedure for drawing definitive conclusions from large bodies of research, found Transcendental Meditation produced a significant increase in basal skin resistance compared to eyes-closed rest, indicating profound relaxation. Deep rest and relaxation were also indicated by greater decreases in respiration rates and plasma lactate levels compared to ordinary rest. These physiological changes occur spontaneously as the mind effortlessly settles to the state of restful alertness, pure consciousness.

Physiological differences between Transcendental Meditation and rest, *American Psychologist* 42: 879–881, 1987.

73

Decreased Stress Hormone

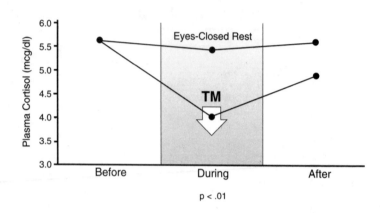

p < .01

Plasma cortisol is a stress hormone. The study shows that plasma cortisol decreased during Transcendental Meditation, whereas it did not change significantly in control subjects during ordinary relaxation.

Adrenocortical activity during meditation, *Hormones and Behavior* 10(1): 54–60, 1978.

Lower Blood Pressure

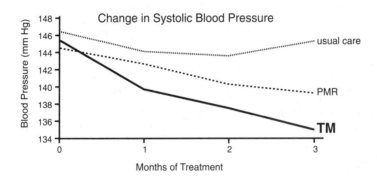

In a clinical experiment with elderly African Americans (mean age 66) dwelling in an inner-city community, Transcendental Meditation was compared with the most widely used method of producing physiological relaxation. Subjects who had moderately elevated blood pressure levels were randomly assigned Transcendental Meditation, Progressive Muscle Relaxation (PMR), or usual care. Over a 3-month interval, systolic and diastolic blood pressure dropped by 10.6 and 5.9 mm Hg, respectively, in the Transcendental Meditation group, and 4.0 and 2.1. mm Hg in the PMR group, with virtually no change in the usual care group. A second random assignment study with the elderly conducted at Harvard found similar blood pressure changes produced by Transcendental Meditation over 3 months (11 mm Hg for systolic blood pressure).

Reference I: In search of an optimal behavioral treatment for hypertension: A review and focus on Transcendental Meditation, chapter in *Personality, Elevated Blood Pressure, and Essential Hypertension* (Washington, D.C., Hemisphere Publishing, 1992). **Reference II:** Transcendental Meditation, mindfulness, and longevity: An experimental study with the elderly, *Journal of Personality and Social Psychology* 57(6): 950–964, 1989.

"More bounce in my step. Good health. Good humor. Good relations. I enjoy my church more. I haven't been to a doctor—except to take life insurance exams—since I started meditating 22 years ago."

—Sam Marasco, Sr., 67, Advertising Sales Manager at the San Diego Sports Arena, San Diego. Thirty-three members of Mr. Marasco's extended family have learned Transcendental Meditation, including his 95-year-old mother-in-law, Grandma Macri.

Reversal of the Aging Process

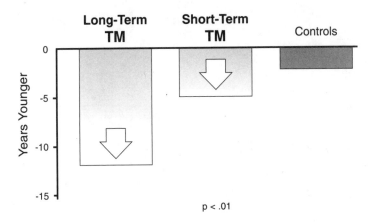

p < .01

Biological age measures how old a person is physiologically. As a group, long-term meditators who had been practicing Transcendental Meditation for more than 5 years were physiologically 12 years younger than their chronological age, as measured by reduction of blood pressure, and better near-point vision and auditory discrimination. Short-term meditators were physiologically 5 years younger than their chronological age. The study controlled for the effects of diet and exercise.

The Effects of the Transcendental Meditation and TM-Sidhi program on the aging process, *International Journal of Neuroscience* 16 (1): 53–58, 1982.

Reduced Need for Medical Care

Decreased Hospitalization

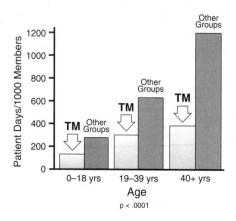

p < .0001

A study of health insurance statistics on over 2,000 people practicing the Transcendental Meditation program over a 5-year period found that the Transcendental Meditation meditators consistently had less than half the hospitalization than did other groups with comparable age, gender, profession, and insurance terms. The difference between the Transcendental Meditation and non-Transcendental Meditation groups increased in older-age brackets. In addition, the Transcendental Meditation meditators had fewer incidents of illness in 17 medical treatment categories, including 87% less hospitalization for heart disease and 55% less for cancer.

Reference I: Medical care utilization and the Transcendental Meditation program, *Psychosomatic Medicine* 49: 493–507, 1987. **Reference II:** Reduced health care utilization in Transcendental Meditation practitioners, presented at the conference of the Society for Behavioral Medicine, Washington, D.C., March 22, 1987.

Reduced Need for Medical Care

**Decreased
Doctor Visits**

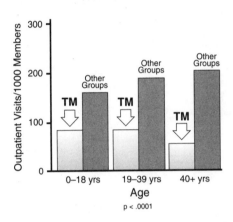

A study of health insurance statistics on over 2,000 people practicing the Transcendental Meditation program over a 5-year period found that the Transcendental Meditation meditators consistently had more than 50% fewer doctor visits than did other groups with comparable age, gender, profession, and insurance terms. The difference between the Transcendental Meditation and non-Transcendental Meditation groups increased in older-age brackets.

Reference I: Medical care utilization and the Transcendental Meditation program, *Psychosomatic Medicine* 49: 493–507, 1987. **Reference II:** Reduced health care utilization in Transcendental Meditation practitioners, presented at the conference of the Society for Behavioral Medicine, Washington, D.C., March 22, 1987.

CHAPTER 4

Ideal Relationships

Bruce Brooks is a versatile and prolific award-winning author who has written 11 books—5 novels and 6 non-fiction—in 10 years. He has won the national Newbery Honor for two of his children's books, and he recently completed a sports biography and a collection of essays on fatherhood. Bruce travels throughout the country, giving several hundred presentations a year, to children, teachers, librarians, and parents, on reading and writing—how to use literature in education and for personal enrichment.

Bruce's wife, Penelope, is an accomplished artist, housewife, and mother of their 10-year-old son, Alex, and their 16-month-old son, Spencer. Penelope does three-dimensional art work in sculpture and lighting, and for several years she taught art and was assistant art director at the Jewish Community Center in the Greater Washington, D.C. area.

Bruce and Penelope have been married 16 years. They live in Silver Spring, Maryland.

Bruce: "I remember the introductory lecture that I attended on Transcendental Meditation. The teacher said, 'When two people come together and both expect to get, then neither receives. When two people come together and both are ready to give, then both receive.'

"Transcendental Meditation allows you to discover just how vast an amount you have to give. You become more secure in yourself by discovering how big you really are; that, in fact, you are infinite. You can give and give and give and you will never exhaust yourself. In my experience that is the secret of relationships, and that has been the secret to raising our children—the capacity for complete giving. And just as you practice Transcendental Meditation as the basis for action, for bringing more of yourself into your work, so, too, in a relationship, you meditate as the basis for bringing more of yourself into the relationship. Only by giving more will you receive more."

Penelope: "Transcendental Meditation has allowed me to experience the depth of love that's within me. It has allowed me to become more aware of my own feelings, desires, and needs, so that I am able to relate more clearly to the feelings, desires, and needs of others. You can only relate to other people—your husband, your children, your friends—based on how you relate to yourself. If you have love in your heart, but your love is buried under stress, it's lost. Since I've been practicing Transcendental Meditation, I've found that love has become a continuum in my life—and not just on certain days, like holidays or birthdays. The love within me comes up and supports me and my activities all the time."

"A strong mind is tolerant; a weak mind is easily overcome by the surroundings."—*Maharishi*

The World Is as You Are

It's a common experience: One morning you wake up as tired as when you went to sleep. The day moves slowly; complications arise; problems seem to be overwhelming. You feel worried; relationships suffer.

But the next morning, after a deep sleep, you feel fresh and alert. The circumstances of the previous day may remain the same, but your evaluation of them differs dramatically. You are more relaxed, yet more energetic, more productive. Relationships are smoother, more harmonious.

Why the difference? Basically, it's because the world is as you are. Put on green glasses and everything appears green. Put on yellow glasses and everything is yellow. Look through tired eyes with an anxious mind and your vision is clouded with problems, many of which, in reality, may not exist.

Look through fresh eyes with an alert, creative mind and you are better able to see solutions to the problems that do exist. When you are rested and fresh, you have the stability, adaptability, energy and intelligence to solve problems and make improvements in all areas of your life.

What's needed? A fully developed consciousness.

Good Social Behavior

In his book *Science of Being and Art of Living,* Maharishi writes, "Really good social behavior between people will only be possible when their awareness is broadened, when they are able to see the whole situation, to understand each other more thoroughly, to be aware of each other's need and attempt to fulfill that need. This naturally necessitates a fully developed consciousness, a right sense of judgement, and all the qualities that only a strong and clear mind possesses."

And without this developed consciousness?

"Small minds always fail to perceive the whole situation and in their narrow vision create imaginary obstacles that are neither useful to themselves nor to anyone else," Maharishi writes. "Then their behavior towards others only results in misunderstanding and increase of tension."

Relationships Thrive on Giving

It's also a common experience that relationships thrive on giving. At home it's the father giving time and attention to his children. At work it's the manager giving enough supervision and support to the sales staff.

But we can only give from what we have. The father who returns home from work exhausted can hardly give his children the love and help they need. Likewise, the manager who is anxious and short-tempered can hardly give the necessary patience and insight to properly train his staff.

What is the solution?

Transcendental Meditation and Relationships

It's a matter of common sense to understand how Maharishi's Transcendental Meditation can improve relationships.

If you're able to think more clearly, you'll be better able to properly evaluate situations and circumstances as they arise. With broader vision you'll be naturally more understanding and patient.

Because you have an effective way to eliminate stress and develop your own unlimited potential, you'll be more fulfilled within yourself, and you won't suffer from the build-up of tension and fatigue. The result? More happiness, less worry, more energy, and a fuller heart. Relationships spontaneously improve, and life naturally becomes much more enjoyable, much more satisfying.

Ralph and Diane Gumps have been married for 38 years. Ralph and Diane and their two grown daughters, Sarah and Julie, learned Transcendental Meditation in Madison, Wisconsin. Ralph is a learning coordinator at Black Hawk Middle School in Madison; Diane is a homemaker; Sarah is married and has gone back to college; and Julie is a senior at the University of Wisconsin, majoring in ecology wildlife. The Gumps have been meditating for one year.

Diane: "Right after learning Transcendental Meditation, I noticed that we were able to communicate better with each other—the edges of things were softer. We've always had a good time together as a we're able to say more things to each other."

Julie: "I used to be so negative, especially coming out of my teenage years. Interacting with friends, we didn't have anything to talk about unless it was, 'Life is terrible.' I am a lot more positive now—less judgemental and more patient with people. Studying goes more quickly now, too. I absorb more information a lot faster. And when I go into a test and don't know the information right away, I don't freeze up as I used to. I can sit back and think it through. That's something new for me. It's been very easy to find time to meditate at school. There have been many times when I've postponed studying for 20 minutes—even though I had a test the next day—so I could meditate. I would never miss it, because it helps me so much."

Ralph: "I think the interactions with my wife and daughters are much better, much easier, since we've been meditating. We always had a good relationship, but now we are able to tell each other things that are accepted in a more positive way. In addition, my physical check-up was better. My blood pressure always used to run a little high, but this year it was down, and I hadn't taken any medication for it."

Diane: "I was always the anxious type. I had this free-floating anxiety, butterflies in my stomach. The first thing I noticed after learning Transcendental Meditation was that the anxiety left. I am much calmer now. I've also seen definite changes in my husband. He has a very stressful job. There's quite a bit of difference in him now when he comes home from work. He's more relaxed; he's a lot easier around the house. And I also think he has a lot easier time at work.

"We look forward to life more each day. We see fewer things as problems. We have a growing sense of 'We can handle this, whatever comes along.'"

The following charts are just a few of the research studies on the effects of Transcendental Meditation for reducing anxiety, increasing self-esteem and self-actualization, as well as for reducing substance abuse.

Reduced Anxiety

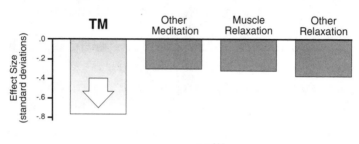

p < .001

A statistical meta-analysis conducted at Stanford University of all available studies—146 independent outcomes—indicated that the effect of the Transcendental Meditation program on reducing anxiety as a character trait was much greater than that of all other meditation and relaxation techniques, including muscle relaxation. This analysis also showed that the positive Transcendental Meditation result could not be attributed to subject expectation, experimenter bias, or quality of research design.

Differential effects of relaxation techniques on trait anxiety: A meta-analysis, *Journal of Clinical Psychology* 45: 957–974, 1989.

Increased Self-Actualization

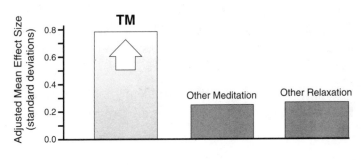

p = .0002

Self-actualization refers to realizing more of one's inner potential, expressed in every area of life. A statistical meta-analysis of all available studies—of 42 independent studies—indicated that the effect of Transcendental Meditation on increasing self-actualization is markedly greater than that of other forms of meditation and relaxation. This analysis statistically controlled for length of treatment and quality of research design.

Transcendental Meditation, self-actualization, and psychological health: A conceptual overview and statistical meta-analysis, *Journal of Social Behavior and Personality* 6: 189–248, 1991.

"I am comfortable and secure within myself, no matter what is happening around me, and because of that my effectiveness has multipled many times. There is no amount of money for which I would give up all I have gained from this remarkably simple practice. It is a priceless treasure."

—Jonathon D. Levy, Assistant Dean, School of Industrial and Labor Relations, Cornell University, Ithaca, New York.

Increased Strength of Self-Concept

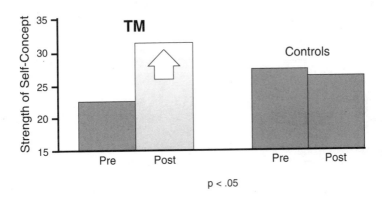

p < .05

One month after beginning Transcendental Meditation, subjects experienced an improved self-concept in comparison to before learning the technique. Transcendental Meditation participants developed a more strongly defined self-concept and also came to perceive their "actual self" as significantly closer to their "ideal self." No similar changes were observed for matched controls.

Reference I: Effects of Transcendental Meditation on self-identity indices and personality, *British Journal of Psychology* 73: 57–68, 1982.
Reference II: Psychological research on the effects of the Transcendental Meditation technique on a number of personality variables, *Gedrag: Tijdschrift voor Psychologie (Behavior: Journal of Psychology)* 4: 206–218, 1976.

Decreased Cigarette, Alcohol, and Drug Abuse

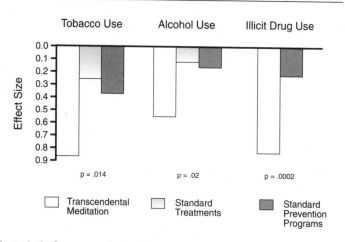

A statistical meta-analysis of 198 independent treatment outcomes found that Transcendental Meditation produced a significantly larger reduction in tobacco, alcohol, and illicit drug use than either standard substance abuse treatments (including counseling, pharmacological treatments, relaxation training, and Twelve-step programs) or prevention programs (such as programs to counteract peer-pressure and promote personal development). This meta-analysis controlled for strength of study design and included both heavy and casual users. Whereas the effects of conventional programs typically decrease sharply by 3 months, effects of Transcendental Meditation on total abstinence from tobacco, alcohol, and illicit drug ranged from 51%–89% over an 18–22 month period.

Reference I: Treating and preventing alcohol, nicotine, and drug abuse through Transcendental Meditation: A review and statistical meta-analysis, *Alcoholism Treatment Quarterly* 11: 13-87, 1994. **Reference II:** Effectiveness of the Transcendental Meditation program in preventing and treating substance misuse: A review, *International Journal of the Addictions* 26: 293-325, 1991.

"Substance abuse disorders are no longer a black or Hispanic or poor problem. They are now everyone's problem. You can go to the best university campuses in this country, and you will find a large percentage of kids strung out on alcohol and drugs. That's a fact. It's a nationwide disaster. The very fabric of what constitutes the future of any society, which is the integrated mental and physical health of all its members—especially its youth—it is actually being torn to pieces right now from coast to coast.

"As someone who has treated thousands of people who have suffered from the disease of substance abuse, I cannot make a stronger recommendation than this: The government should research Transcendental Meditation, understand it, and put it into practice immediately as part of a relapse prevention program. Society cannot afford to overlook the power that Transcendental Meditation can bring for healing the horrible disease that now plagues us—violence and drug abuse. Transcendental Meditation is easy to learn, effective, and cost effective, and the time has come for it to be used and understood."

—Marcelino Cruces, LICSW, has supervised substance-abuse treatment programs for over 15 years in Washington, D.C. and Los Angeles. He has served as a consultant for the development of protocols for the treatment of alcohol, drug abuse, and mental health disorders for the U.S. Department of Health and Human Services and the U.S. State Department. He is a member of the District of Columbia Mayor's Advisory Committee on Drug Abuse and is chief administrator for the Coalition of Latino Community-Based Organizations and clinical director of the Salud Health Center in the District of Columbia.

CHAPTER 5

Promoting Corporate Development

R.W. "Buck" Montgomery, Jr., wanted to turn around his Detroit-based chemical manufacturing company, the H.A. Montgomery Company.

"The company had been in business for over 40 years," Buck recalls. "It had gotten into a routine, a rut of old-time management, and it was difficult to get the people to see new thinking. That was in 1983, and at the time the U.S. automotive industry was in a great slump, stalled by imports from Japan and Germany.

"We needed a new approach to everything—a new attitude, new thinking, new energy to revitalize the company and get it to take off again."

Buck and his staff attended numerous seminars and courses.

"We would go to weekend or week-long seminars, and we'd return with these huge books, and we'd still be plagued with the same problems. We'd forget what we learned, or we didn't have time to restudy what we'd learned, due to the demands of the job, and so we just went back to our old routine.

"I was looking for a tool that my employees could

utilize every day, that would allow them to change their thinking, allow them to have more energy, be more creative on their own, and use more of their potential on the job. I found Transcendental Meditation to be the tool that would work."

Buck sat down with his senior staff and came up with a plan. First, Transcendental Meditation would be offered at company expense to anyone interested among the managers. They would meditate twice a day for 6 months. They would be asked, on a monthly basis, to write progress reports, pro or con, on what they thought of the program and how it was affecting them in their daily life—both at the office and at home. Then they would decide if the program would go company-wide.

"After 6 months there was 100% agreement among that management group to offer the program throughout the company," Buck says. "Transcendental Meditation was then introduced into research, manufacturing, sales, marketing, and administration."

Buck encouraged his managers and employees to meditate at least once a day—in the morning or in the late afternoon—on company time at the plant.

"Productivity improved dramatically," Buck says. "Absenteeism decreased drastically, as did sick days and injuries. The creativity of our research department went up, sales increased 120% in 2 years, and profitability went up 520%."

In 1987 Buck sold the company and retired. He now spends his time with his family and consults with companies that are looking for new avenues for success. He is often asked to speak on the success of the Transcendental Meditation program at the former H.A. Montgomery Company to executives who are interested in repeating that success in their own firms.

"The individual is the most important resource a business has," Buck says. "You've got to improve the capacity and capabilities of the individual. If you take a tired individual, or one who is not motivated or who doesn't feel he has any creativity, no matter what tools you put in his hands, it's a waste of time. First you have to improve the individual, increase his potential; then you can give him other tools to work with. The only program that I know that will do that is Transcendental Meditation. The small amount of money it costs today will be of immeasurable benefit to the company on the profitability line and on a morale line—and everything else you can imagine. This is success."

U.S. business is being crippled by stress. Up to $200 billion is lost—wasted, actually—each year due to stress in the work place, according to a 1993 report by the United Nations International Labor Organization.

Worse yet, research indicates that none of the programs for stress reduction/personal development widely in use in business and industry today provide a solution to the problem. Despite intensive efforts to curb the impact of stress in the work place, medical care utilization costs continue to escalate, and job performance, productivity, and employee turnover rates continue to suffer.

"In this era of increased competition and downsizing, businesses have asked people to do more and more work in less and less time," says Gerald Swanson, Ph.D., Professor of Management at Maharishi International University, who has introduced Transcendental Meditation in several U.S. corporations and has written a book, *Enlightened Management,* on the use of the technique in business. "This puts more stress on the employees and leaves them burned out and unable to have a good time with their families.

"Today most people in business are looking for some way to re-establish the balance between home and work. They are torn between the need to maintain their financial stability and security and the need to come home and nurture their family. This is especially true now that there is such a large number of two-career marriages and single-parent families. Both the mom and the dad are being called upon to be bread winners and still provide that nurturing value to their family.

"How can you do that unless you have some way of not being overwhelmed by the stress of working? The only way to do that is to have a stronger, more resilient physiology.

"We know from research and experiences in business that that's precisely how people feel when they practice Transcendental Meditation," Dr. Swanson says.

A Cost-Effective Solution to Job Stress

In the past 36 years, Maharishi's Transcendental Meditation has been learned by tens of thousands of business professionals. The technique has also been offered company-wide to executives, managers, and employees in hundreds of large corporations and small businesses throughout the world.

Scientific research in several of these business settings has found that Transcendental Meditation offers a cost-effective solution to problems caused by job stress. The research shows that sickness, absenteeism, and health care utilization decrease; productivity and job satisfaction improve; and relationships between co-workers and supervisors improve.

Transcendental Meditation in a Fortune 100 Company

For example, a study published in the scientific journal *Anxiety, Stress and Coping* in December 1993 found significant benefits of Transcendental Meditation in stress reduction, health, and employee development, in two companies.

Managers and employees in a large manufacturing plant of a Midwest Fortune 100 company and in a smaller Pennsylvania sales distribution company learned the technique.

After 3 months employees who learned Transcendental Meditation were compared to a control group of non-meditating employees who worked at similar job sites, held similar job positions, and had similar demographics (age, education, etc.) and similar personality characteristics, before the study began.

Researchers found that compared to controls, the Transcendental Meditation group had significantly

- Less anxiety, job tension, insomnia, and fatigue
- Reduced cigarette and hard liquor use
- Improved health and fewer health complaints
- Enhanced effectiveness, job satisfaction, and work/personal relationships

The research showed that the effects of Transcendental Meditation on anxiety, alcohol and cigarette use, and in enhancing personal development, were much larger than for other forms of meditation and relaxation found in previous studies.

Worry over the negative impact of rising job stress led employees at Puritan-Bennett Corporation, the world's leading maker of respiratory care products, to ask the company to address the problem.

"We researched the best stress-reduction/personal development programs," says Dr. Mary Martha Stevens, Manager of Health and Wellness at Puritan-Bennett. "We decided on Transcendental Meditation for three reasons: The technique had the most research supporting it; the best follow-up of any program of its type; and clearly from what I had discovered, it was the easiest, most practical, and most effective technique for busy individuals to use."

Puritan-Bennett offered the Transcendental Meditation Corporate Development Program at its corporate headquarters in Kansas City in August 1993. Sixty-six managers and employees and ten spouses learned the technique during the program's first phase. Instruction was held on company time, as was a complete 4-month follow-up program. For those with work schedule problems, instruction was also held after hours.

The benefits were immediate, according to Dr. Stevens. After just a few days, managers reported that they felt more relaxed and less anxious, were thinking more clearly, and were able to organize themselves better and accomplish much more.

Diana Trompeter is payroll supervisor for the Puritan Group at Puritan-Bennett. She has been with the company for 13 years. Diana learned Transcendental Meditation because she had been under extreme stress from the death of her mother and increasing pressures at work. After 4 weeks of practicing the technique, Diana wrote a letter to Dr. Stevens, assessing her progress:

"In the beginning I wasn't sure what TM would do for me, and when I shared the idea with my staff, they had doubts, too. I decided to try it, and it is one of my best decisions.

"TM immediately changed things for me. I became calm and clear-minded after my first session, and it works as well for me now, 4 weeks later, as it did that first day. TM is one of the few things that is truly effortless and yet you can see the benefit.

"My employees have commented on the difference in me and in other meditators they often work with. Of all the good benefits the company has offered us through the years, this is by far the most beneficial for me. I feel better, more confident about my decisions, and most important, I feel a peace and calm that seems to get me through the most difficult times.

"Thank you for introducing TM to us, and I would like to see it offered to all our employees."

Ten months after learning the technique, Diana reported that the benefits were continuing to grow.

"Transcendental Meditation has produced a calmness and serenity in me that allows me to deal with my job and the people around me in a much more pleasant and efficient manner. Nothing outside of me has changed. The job pressures are still there; the problems are still there. Transcendental Meditation is simply a way of letting me handle my own life better so that I am better at dealing with those outside pressures. It is the best thing I have ever done."

In the project design a research component was included to evaluate objectively the effects of the program on 38 meditating executives compared with 38 matched controls. The findings: Over a 3-month period, the meditators reduced psychological and physical symptoms of stress, reduced total blood cholesterol, gained vitality, and enhanced mental health and well-being.

Dr. Stevens said that Puritan-Bennett was very satisfied with the results and that she strongly recommends Transcendental Meditation to other companies. "If you want your employees to eliminate stress and not just cope with it—which is what companies spend a great deal of time doing today—then having them learn Transcendental Meditation is the best way to do it."

The following charts are just a few of the research studies on the effects of Transcendental Meditation for improving productivity and relationships, reducing stress, and promoting health, on the job.

Increased Productivity

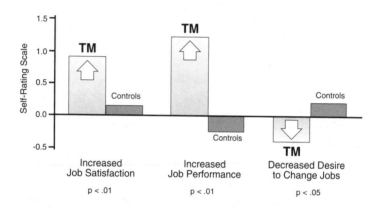

In this study subjects practicing the Transcendental Meditation program showed significant improvements at work, compared with members of a control group. Job performance and job satisfaction increased while desire to change jobs decreased. People at every level of the organization benefited from practicing the Transcendental Meditation program.

Transcendental Meditation and productivity, *Academy of Management Journal* 17 (2): 362–368, 1974.

Improved Relations at Work

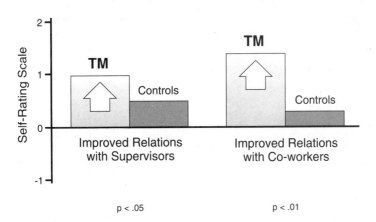

Transcendental Meditation and productivity, *Academy of Management Journal* 17 (2): 362–368, 1974.

This study found significant improvements in relations with supervisors and co-workers after an average of 11 months practicing Transcendental Meditation, in comparison to control subjects. And while Transcendental Meditation practitioners reported that they felt less anxiety about promotion (shown by reduced climb orientation), their fellow employees saw them as moving ahead quickly. People at every level of the organization benefited from practicing the Transcendental Meditation program.

Increased Relaxation and Decreased Stress

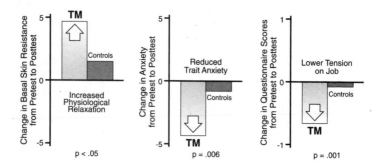

This 3-month study of managers and employees who regularly practiced the Transcendental Meditation technique in a Fortune 100 manufacturing company and a smaller distribution-sales company showed that Transcendental Meditation practitioners displayed more relaxed physiological functioning, a greater reduction in anxiety, and reduced tension on the job, when compared to control subjects with similar job positions in the same companies.

A prospective study of the effects of the Transcendental Meditation program in two business settings, *Anxiety, Stress and Coping: International Journal* 6: 245–262, 1993.

Improved Health and More Positive Health Habits

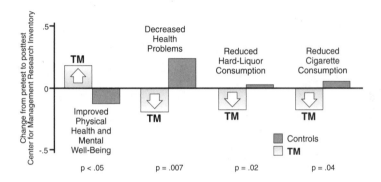

In 2 companies that introduced the Transcendental Meditation program, managers and employees who regularly practiced Transcendental Meditation improved significantly in overall physical health, mental well-being, and vitality when compared to control subjects with similar jobs in the same companies. Transcendental Meditation practitioners also reported significant reductions in health problems such as headaches and backaches, improved quality of sleep, and a significant reduction in the use of hard liquor and cigarettes, compared to personnel in control groups.

A prospective study of the effects of the Transcendental Meditation program in two business settings, *Anxiety, Stress and Coping: International Journal* 6: 245–262, 1993.

CHAPTER 6

Life Supported
by Natural Law

"The more years that I meditate, the smoother my life goes, and the more good luck, the more support I get in my activity from the environment and from people around me," says Fred Gratzon, chairman of Telegroup, Inc., a long distance international discount carrier. Founded in 1989, Telegroup is now one of the fastest growing companies in America. The firm has clients in 114 countries.

"Transcendental Meditation refines my thinking and feelings so that I am more in tune with the subtle creative impulses deep within me—and to the source of those creative impulses. When I am in tune with that, I have very good luck. It's as simple as that. It's an abstract thing to describe, but it's a very real experience. When I have it I feel confident. It's like an athlete who is in the 'zone.' I want the ball. I know I'll hit the shot. I can't miss. That's a metaphor for everything in my life. I feel that I've got the rhythm, I'm hot. I have come to expect support of nature, even insist upon it. And I know what I have to do to keep it. I meditate. Everyone in business should have this experience. No, *everyone* should have it."

"If you favor natural law, natural law will favor you."—*Maharishi*

Support of Natural Law for Success in Life

One day everything is a strain. You feel worried and tense and out of-step with the day. You just miss an important phone call, hit all the red lights when you're rushing for an appointment, and can't find a parking place anywhere.

Another day you feel quite good. Everything seems to go right and click into place. You find the perfect parking place, reach the right person on the phone, and come up with a workable solution to a problem at the office. The day seems to go effortlessly and you wonder why every day can't go at least as smoothly.

It can—through "support of natural law."

Here's how.

What Is a Law of Nature?

Throw a tennis ball up in the air and it falls to the earth: gravity, a law of nature.

Heat water to 212°F and it boils: a law of nature.

Water a plant, give it proper food and sunlight and it grows: laws of nature.

The entire world, the entire universe is governed by laws of nature. Everywhere we look—at DNA through an electron microscope or at the galactic life through a high-powered telescope—everything in the universe is permeated by intelligence; all activity is governed by natural law.

What Is the Purpose of Natural Law?

Like a strong current in a river, natural law propels life in an evolutionary direction. It is the invincible force in nature from the level of the unified field that continually creates, maintains, and evolves life.

Natural Law and You

What does natural law have to do with you? Everything—because not only are electrons and galaxies subject to the laws of nature, but so are you.

There are, for example, countless laws of nature that govern the functioning of your body. If you align yourself with those laws—eat the right foods, exercise properly, get enough rest, etc.—your body maintains its health.

Violate those laws and you fall sick and suffer.

Therefore, the key to better health—actually the key to perfect health—is to attune yourself with all the laws of nature that naturally promote growth and evolution. It's also the key to skill in action in life.

How can that be accomplished?

You Can't *Try* to Live in Accord with Natural Law

Living in accord with natural law is simple through Transcendental Meditation, and we'll see how in a moment. But first, let's analyze the ways that you can't gain this alliance:

• By trying intellectually to understand or remember all of the different laws of nature that govern life;

• By trying strictly to adhere to specific laws of nature.

Why? Because there are far too many laws of nature to understand, much less remember. And, even if you were able to gain some knowledge about specific laws of nature, it's no guarantee you'll be able to abide by them.

For example, there's the medical doctor, a noted authority in the causes of stress-related diseases, who nevertheless gets sick from overwork and worry. He's fully aware of the causes and consequences of stress, yet he is unable to follow his own professional advice. He works too long and too hard.

Or the factory supervisor with a heart condition who's placed on a strict diet and exercise program by his physician. How long does it take before he begins to compromise on his regimen even though it's in his own best interest to maintain it?

What is the difficulty?

To act in a way that is completely life supporting is next to impossible, unless it is natural. It can never be accomplished by trying to remember what's right, or by forcing oneself to behave in a certain way.

Alliance with Natural Law Must Be Spontaneous

Alliance with natural law must be spontaneous. And it can be lived only on the basis of a fully developed consciousness.

Maharishi's Transcendental Meditation places life in the center stream of the evolutionary power of natural law.

How? By allowing the conscious mind to settle down to its most silent, wakeful, and fully expanded state, Transcendental Meditation opens the awareness to pure consciousness, which is the unified field of *all* the laws of nature.

As we discussed earlier, it is the unified field, through its "self-interacting dynamics," which expresses itself as all the diversified forms and phenomena in creation. This means that all matter, all energy, and all the laws of nature that govern all the activity in the universe spring from the unified field.

Concrete, Natural, and Practical

When you open your awareness to the unified field during Transcendental Meditation, you draw upon the unlimited potential of nature at its source. Your mind naturally becomes clearer and more creative. Your body becomes healthier and more energetic. Your thoughts, feelings, and actions are *spontaneously* more in tune with the evolutionary power of natural law. And then you enjoy more success and satisfaction in everything you do.

Does it sound abstract?

It's actually concrete, natural, and very practical.

"I believe that you get back what you give," says Michael Reed, Ph.D., manager in business development for Glaxo Inc., a pharmaceutical company in Research Triangle Park, near Raleigh, in North Carolina. "Transcendental Meditation has allowed me to give more, do more, and live and enjoy my life more fully. At the same time, because I meditate I feel that I am having a positive influence on the people I live with, the people I work with, and society in general.

"Some people just call it good luck, but since I've been meditating I've found that spontaneously good things happen, often without any directed thought or effort on my part. Nature spontaneously delivers opportunities and situations to enhance my job, my family, and my social life.

"I have a wonderful life. I have a beautiful wife, a new baby, a job that is very satisfying, and I live very comfortably. I feel that I'm living the fruits of support of nature every day in many, many ways."

"Everyone has had this happen: You want something and suddenly 5 minutes later, or a day later, it's there and you didn't seem to do anything," says Channler Drawdy, chairman and part-owner of Atherton Technology, a computer-aided software engineering company in Fremont, California. "Most people think this kind of good luck is coincidental, but it doesn't have to be that way. Since I've been practicing Transcendental Meditation these things are occurring with more and more frequency in my business and in my personal life. The amount of support I seem to be spontaneously receiving has reached the point where I can no longer say it's a coincidence. I am able to do less and accomplish more. Life has become simpler and much more enjoyable."

Before acquiring controlling interest in Atherton Technology in 1993, Mr. Drawdy was a software engineering director for Sun Microsystems. Atherton Technology had not been successful since its founding in 1986, but the company turned a profit the first year after Mr. Drawdy and his associates came in. Now we're into an explosive growth period," he says. "We're really taking off fast."

"In my experience, success comes from support of nature. There are laws of nature, like the laws of physics, and you can either violate those laws or you can live in harmony with them. If you live in harmony with those laws, then every aspect of your life is fuller, richer, more successful. If you violate them, then you experience a lot of pain and failure and discomfort. The easiest, fastest way to cultivate harmony with the laws of nature is through Transcendental Meditation."

Solution to Problems Is Alliance with Natural Law

Why do people violate the laws of nature?

"Education is responsible," Maharishi has said. "No educational system in the world is capable of training an individual to function spontaneously in accord with natural law. This lack in education is the cause of all problems in every area of life."

The solution to all problems then, as Maharishi has said, is spontaneous alliance with natural law. Why? Because when you closely examine them, all problems in life originate from the violation of natural law. It is violation of natural law that causes stress. Stress in an individual's life is the cause of sickness and suffering, and the build-up of stress among all the individuals in society is the cause of crime, violence, conflict, and war.

On the other hand, life spontaneously lived in harmony with natural law is the basis for a healthy, prosperous, and fulfilling life for the individual, and the foundation for lasting peace and progress for the whole world.

CHAPTER 7

Reducing Crime in Society and Creating World Peace

"We are in a highly stressed area, an area that has a lot of drugs and a lot of violence," says Dr. George Rutherford, Principal of the Fletcher-Johnson School in southeast Washington, D.C. There are 840 students in grades pre-K through 9, and 125 staff at the school. Dr. Rutherford has been practicing Transcendental Meditation for 2 years.

"Some of my students and former students have been shot; some of my former students have been killed. That brings about tremendous stress in me because I know these kids, and I have to worry that my school is safe for my students and staff. I have to make sure that I don't have the outside forces coming in. In order to do that I've got to be able to think clearly enough to run my building and still try to assure youngsters that this is a safe haven.

"Transcendental Meditation is the best thing I have ever done to help myself. I have more energy. I am less stressful. I can think clearer, and I believe I have become a better principal. My tolerance level is higher, so I am able to talk clearer to youngsters and understand the things that are affecting them.

"My health is outstanding. If I had not started Transcendental Meditation, I'd have left the school system or I'd be dead because of all the pressure. It has made me much stronger physically and much stronger mentally.

"I truly feel that Transcendental Meditation is a vehicle that we can use to reduce or eliminate the violence in our community. It will help to remove all the baggage that young people bring to school with them that makes them ready to jump and fight at the first moment anyone touches them. If they can meditate at home, it will help them remove the stresses that they have each and every day—and that is from hearing gunshots at night and seeing people get killed—family members and friends. Transcendental Meditation is going to eventually remove that kind of behavior.

"I would whole-heartedly support large groups of Transcendental Meditation meditators in Washington to reduce crime and create peace in the community. Nothing else has worked. I feel, based on my experience with Transcendental Meditation, that this is the means, the vehicle that is going to get us to a peaceful society. The government should support these large groups, if, in fact, it is serious about reducing or eliminating crime."

"Only a new seed can yield a new crop. Only new knowledge, new principles, and new programs can put an end to conflict, sickness, and suffering, and prevent such problems from arising in the future. Only new knowledge can create a healthy, prosperous, harmonious society and a peaceful world."

—*Maharishi*

The Problems of Violence

Crime spreads at an alarming rate through our cities. Regional conflicts rage in many parts of the globe.

Billions of dollars urgently needed for education, health care, etc., are allocated to build more prisons and hire more police, but no one is safe from the threat of rising violent crime.

Peacekeeping forces are sent, at considerable risk and expense, to far-off lands to quell conflicts. Experienced diplomats hammer out peace accords between opposing factions. Yet order is not maintained, and lasting peace is not delivered.

Nothing is working. What's wrong?

The Cause of Crime and War

What's wrong, according to Maharishi, is that the root cause of violence—both in crime and war—has not been addressed. Both are the outburst of built-up stress in society. And stress in society is created by all the people in society continually violating the laws of nature.

119

"As long as individuals continue to violate the laws of nature, they will continue to create stress in their own lives and create stress in the collective consciousness of the whole nation," Maharishi says. "As a result, governmental efforts to promote peace will prove ineffective, and the world will face violence and conflict everywhere. Peace will only remain an abstract, unattainable ideal."

Old Approaches Fail to Reduce Stress in Society

Like smokestacks pouring pollution into the atmosphere, individuals suffering from stress pour stress into the environment, creating the ground for crime, violence, and conflict in society.

The approaches that have been tried repeatedly—more police, longer prison terms, military force, peace agreements—have ultimately failed because they fail to solve the problem of high levels of stress in society.

A New Seed for a New Crop

Only a new seed can yield a new crop. A completely new approach is needed that can reduce the dangerous rise of stress and crime in our cities and, at the same time, reduce the dangerous rise of stress and conflict in the world's trouble spots.

Fortunately, such an approach exists. It has been developed during the past 36 years, and it has been found to work. What follows is a brief explanation of this approach, including a history of its development, a discussion of its mechanics, and the research that shows that it works.

Individual Is the Basic Unit of World Peace

When Maharishi first started teaching Transcendental Meditation in 1958, he said that the technique was a way for the individual to grow in health and happiness, and for the world to rise in peace.

"For the forest to be green, every tree must be green," Maharishi said. "The individual is the basic unit of world peace. For the world to be at peace, every individual has to be at peace."

Maharishi said that Transcendental Meditation was the key to producing a peaceful individual, and therefore was the basis for creating world peace.

One Percent for World Peace

A few years later Maharishi made a prediction: If as little as 1% of the world's population practiced Transcendental Meditation, there would be no more wars. The peaceful influence created by people practicing Transcendental Meditation, he said, radiates throughout the environment, like the light from a bulb radiates throughout a darkened room.

At that time, in the early 1960s, there were too few meditators in the world to test Maharishi's prediction, even on a small scale. But by the end of 1974, more than 250,000 people were meditating in the United States, and many small cities in the country had 1% of their population practicing the technique.

The first study to test Maharishi's prediction occurred in December 1974, when scientists measured quality-of-life indicators in 4 cities where 1% of the population was practicing Transcendental Meditation. They examined such standard and publicly accessible indices as crime statistics, accident rates, and hospital admissions.

Decreased Crime in 1% Cities

When these findings were compared with similar research from four control cities matched for population density, geography, economic conditions, etc., a remarkable discovery was made.

The cities with 1% of their populations practicing the Transcendental Meditation program showed a decrease in crime rate while the matched control cities showed an increase in crime rate—as did the U.S. as a whole.

The researchers then expanded their study to include eleven 1% cities and eleven control cities. They found a 16.6 percent reduction in crime rates among the 1% cities compared to the non-one-percent cities.

What did it mean? It was the first scientific validation of Maharishi's prediction that the quality of life could be improved through a small percentage of a population practicing Transcendental Meditation.

On January 12, 1975, in the presence of leading scientists, doctors, educators, business leaders, and the world press, Maharishi hailed the significance of this discovery by inaugurating "the dawn of the Age of Enlightenment" for the world.

Maharishi said, "With 1% of a city's population

practicing Transcendental Meditation, crime rates decrease. One percent of the world's population practicing the Transcendental Meditation program will neutralize stress and negativity, and promote positivity and peace, throughout the world. With just this first scientific research on the sociological effects of Transcendental Meditation we can see the onset of a new age of progress and harmony for all mankind."

Transcendental Meditation Is the Causal Factor

The research continued. The 11-city study was expanded to include 48 cities, with similar results. The study, entitled "The Transcendental Meditation Program and Crime Rate Change in a Sample of Forty-Eight Cities," was published in the *Journal of Crime and Justice* (Vol. IV, 1981).

Since 1974 Transcendental Meditation crime-rate studies have been conducted in hundreds of cities in the United States, using some of the most sophisticated, computerized, statistical procedures to control for a broad spectrum of variables.

The conclusion: Transcendental Meditation program participation was found to be the causal factor in crime rate reductions in cities and metropolitan areas throughout the nation. Scientists named the effect the "Maharishi Effect."

How is this possible?

We'll see in a moment.

The Transcendental Meditation-Sidhi Program

Concurrent with all of this, a new development was taking place that was to have a profound impact on the direction of Transcendental Meditation research.

In 1976 Maharishi introduced the Transcendental Meditation-Sidhi program, which he described as advanced procedures or natural extensions of Transcendental Meditation "to train consciousness to function from the unified field of natural law, the self-referral state of pure consciousness."

Maharishi explained that the Transcendental Meditation-Sidhi program trained the awareness to function in the same self-interacting style as the intelligence of nature. In this way, Maharishi said, individuals would gain the support of the total potential of nature's creativity and intelligence for the fulfillment of their desires in daily life.

Scientific research showed that Maharishi's Transcendental Meditation-Sidhi program significantly enhanced the benefits of Transcendental Meditation. It increased EEG coherence, increased creativity and intelligence, and promoted longevity.

Most dramatically, sociological research showed that the practice of the Transcendental Meditation-Sidhi program by a small number of people together in one place had a very powerful effect on society as a whole—even more powerful than the 1% Transcendental Meditation effect.

Research showed that only the square root of 1% of a population practicing the Transcendental Meditation-

Sidhi program together in one place was required to create an influence of order and coherence in the entire population.

How is all of this possible? How can people meditating alone in their homes or offices, or together in a group, influence other people across town—or across the country—who aren't even meditating?

The Super Radiance Effect: Action at a Distance

• Two corks are floating in a sink of water 8 inches apart. Push down one cork, release it, and the other cork bobs up and down.

• Turn on the radio as you drive to the supermarket. A disc jockey is playing a song 50 miles away. The music fills your car.

These are two examples where one object can influence another object at a distance. In physics this phenomenon is called "action at a distance."

How does it happen? Through the influence of waves traveling through an underlying field. Water links the two corks, and the electromagnetic field links the radio station and the car radio.

Connecting all matter in the universe are unseen, fundamental fields—the electromagnetic field, the gravitational field, and the fields of the weak and strong forces binding the center of the atom.

At their basis, according to supersymmetric unified quantum field theories, is the unified field, which creates and connects everything together in the universe—all fields, all matter, everything, everybody.

The Behavior of Fields

One interesting characteristic about the behavior of fields is the manner in which waves travel through them.

For example, consider the ordinary light radiating from your reading lamp. It is the product of innumerable light waves that are random and incoherent in their pattern. Take any 100 of these incoherent light waves and they produce the light of 100 separate waves. Because of this the light from your lamp is bright enough for you to read the book in your lap, but not nearly bright enough, say, to reach the moon.

On the other hand, if those random light waves are made coherent so that the peaks and valleys of each wave are in step with each other, then the intensity of the light waves becomes far greater than when they function separately. Their intensity is proportional to the *square* of the actual number of waves. Take those 100 light waves again, make them function coherently together, and they will produce a light as bright as 10,000 incoherent light waves.

Coherent light is called laser light. It can be bounced off the moon, applied to conduct surgery, or used to play a laser disc recording. This phenomenon has been called the "superradiance effect."

The Field Effects of Consciousness

How, then, can the coherence created by a small number of people practicing the Transcendental Meditation and TM-Sidhi program together in one place affect a large population?

Scientists said it could happen only if consciousness, experienced in its self-referral state during Transcendental Meditation, is a field and only if it is the same unified field that underlies all of nature.

They said that only a field can produce the influence of "action-at-a-distance," and only the unified field would be able to account for the wide-ranging effects on society observed with the collective practice of the Transcendental Meditation and TM-Sidhi program. This is because on the level of the unified field, everything in nature is connected.

Researchers predicted that if a group of experts in the Transcendental Meditation and TM-Sidhi program could, in fact, produce an influence of coherence on the level of the unified field, then according to the behavior of fields, that coherence would spread throughout the environment.

That's the hypothesis. Now does it actually happen? What is the evidence? And how can it be measured?

Measuring the Trends of Time

In the past two decades, social scientists have developed sophisticated statistical procedures to analyze changing trends in society. These methods are helpful to researchers attempting to determine why these changes occur.

For example, sickness rates might be found to be suddenly decreasing in a particular city. Why? Is it due to a public health program recently introduced into the school system, or is it simply a seasonal change?

Through these advanced statistical procedures, scientists are better able to identify the reason, or reasons, for the decrease in sickness rates in the city, eliminate alternative explanations, and hopefully use the technology or program to produce the same effect again, perhaps on a wider scale.

Studying the Effects of Transcendental Meditation on Quality of Life

Extensive research, employing many of these statistical procedures, have been conducted throughout the world to gauge the effects of the Transcendental Meditation and TM-Sidhi program on the quality of life in society.

The research has demonstrated repeatedly that when the square root of 1% of a population practices the Transcendental Meditation and TM-Sidhi program together in one place there are marked decreases in negative tendencies such as crime, sickness, and accident rates, as well as instances of turbulence and violence in society. The research has also shown significant increases in positive trends, such as improvements in economic conditions.

7,000 Assembly at Maharishi International University

The largest experiment studying the impact of group practice of the Transcendental Meditation and TM-Sidhi program occurred from December 17, 1983, to January 6, 1984, at Maharishi International University in Fairfield, Iowa.

Seven thousand experts in the Transcendental Meditation and TM-Sidhi program from over 50 nations gathered at the university to create "an upsurge of coherence" for the whole world. Seven thousand is approximately the square root of 1% of the world's population.

The findings confirmed predictions made by scientists in advance. Research showed an immediate increase in positivity in situations of international conflict. Available data from major countries on several continents also showed that traffic fatalities per miles driven and the incidence of infectious diseases dropped during the assembly, while patent applications and other signs of creativity and positivity rose.

And after the assembly? All the positive trends returned to the usual patterns that had characterized them prior to the assembly.

A New Formula for Peace

Based on these findings, as well as on similar results from several other large assemblies throughout the world, Maharishi declared 1987 to the Year of World Peace. He presented a program to reduce crime and violence in society and create peace in the world. Maharishi's plan called for the establishment in every country of a permanent group of 7,000 experts practicing the Transcendental Meditation and TM-Sidhi program together in one place.

Maharishi said that this group would immediately reduce the dangerous build-up of stress in collective consciousness and create "an indomitable influence of coherence and positivity in national and world consciousness to ensure that all political, social, and economic trends will always remain positive and enriching."

For There to Be Peace in Society

Maharishi also laid out a plan whereby every individual can contribute his or her share to promote peace. "For there to be peace in society, there must be peace in the individuals in society," Maharishi said. "Transcendental Meditation is a technique for gaining peace. If you have peace then you should engage in creating world peace by bringing your friends and family to start this practice. Unless you create peace in your family and friends, your own peace will be fragile and world peace will have no meaning for you. With peace in every home in our precious family of nations, Heaven will be created on Earth."

Scientific Research Expands

Research on group practice of the Transcendental Meditation and TM-Sidhi program continued to expand. By 1990 there were over 40 sociological studies, including research showing positive effects on reducing urban crime, decreasing conflict in the Middle East, and reducing violent death. The studies were published in some of America's leading peer-reviewed scientific journals, including *Journal of Conflict Resolution*, *Social Indicators Research*, and *Journal of Mind and Behavior*.

The Urgent Need for a New Solution to Crime

By this time the alarming rise of violent crime in U.S. cities had also made it very clear that a new solution to the crisis was urgently needed. Despite the expenditure of tens of billions of dollars on crime-fighting programs, violent crime continued to soar. Experts admitted that conventional approaches had failed. In fact, there was no evidence to suggest that building more prisons, hiring more police, or handing out stiffer sentences to offenders were making even the slightest dent in reducing crime.

Two-Month Crime Reduction Demonstration Project in Washington, D.C.

There was, however, considerable evidence to show that group practice of the Transcendental Meditation and TM-Sidhi program did reduce violent crime. To demonstrate this fact publicly, a $5 million sociological experiment was held in Washington, D.C., during the summer of 1993.

From June 7 through July 30, 4,000 experts in the Transcendental Meditation and TM-Sidhi program from 50 countries assembled, at their own expense, in Washington, D.C. Twice a day they participated in large group meditations to reduce social stress and violent crime.

Researchers lodged predictions for the experiment in advance with a 27-member, independent "project review board" comprising leading research scientists from universities throughout the U.S., including the University of Maryland, the University of the District of Columbia, and the University of Denver School of Law; policy analysts; and local government and community leaders. Based on previous findings, researchers predicted that violent crime in Washington, D.C., would decrease significantly by the end of the project. In addition, because of reduced levels of stress in the nation's capital, researchers also predicted an increase in the level of cooperation and effectiveness of the government and, on that basis, an improvement in President Clinton's standing in the opinion polls.

Violent Crime in Washington Decreases Significantly during Demonstration

The results exceeded predictions. After months of rapid increase, HRA violent crime (homicide, rape, and assault) suddenly declined in Washington, D.C., during the demonstration, according to time series analysis. (Violent crime usually increases in June and July.) For the final 2 weeks of the demonstration, HRA crime dropped 18%. In addition, other quality-of-life indicators moved in the positive direction, and an analysis of opinion polls on President Clinton showed a highly statistically significant change from a declining trend to a trend of increasing public support during the demonstration. Once the Transcendental Meditation assembly dispersed and social stress began to rise again, HRA crime rose as well. (The results of this study will be expanded and finalized after the District of Columbia Metropolitan Police Department releases its complete crime report for 1993 to the FBI in October 1994—following the publication of this book. For a copy of the final results of the Washington study, contact the Institute of Science, Technology and Public Policy at Maharishi International University, Fairfield, Iowa 52557.)

"This demonstration has confirmed the theory that large assemblies of people practicing the Transcendental Meditation and TM-Sidhi program reduce social stress and tension, as measured by decreased violent crime, increased governmental cooperation and efficiency, and improvements in other sociological indicators," says Dr. John Hagelin, Director of the Institute of Science, Technology and Public Policy at Maharishi International University. "It shows definitively that any government can reduce crime and other social problems, and prevent new problems from arising, by establishing 'A Group for a Government'—a large group of experts practicing the Transcendental Meditation and TM-Sidhi program. Governments now have a practical means to prevent costly problems and dramatically improve the quality of life for the whole population."

"I think the claim can be plausibly made that the potential impact of this research exceeds that of any other on-going social or psychological research program," says David Edwards, Ph.D., Professor of Government at the University of Texas at Austin, referring to the many studies conducted on effects of the Transcendental Meditation and TM-Sidhi program on society. "The research has survived a broader array of statistical tests than has most research in the field of conflict resolution. I think this work, and the theory that informs it, deserve the most serious consideration by academics and policy makers alike." Dr. Edwards does not practice Transcendental Meditation.

"There is growing recognition that we have been thinking too narrowly about the causes, dynamics, and means of resolving conflicts," says John Davies, Ph.D., Research Coordinator for the Center of International Development and Conflict Management at the University of Maryland. "This thinking hasn't given us sufficiently effective options to be able to manage and minimize conflict in the world."

Dr. Davies is an expert on the prevention, analysis, and resolution of conflict. He is currently developing the most advanced and sophisticated global event data system for tracking daily international and intra-national events worldwide. International peace-keeping organizations will use the data system for developing early warning systems and evaluating the success of attempts to prevent or resolve conflicts.

Dr. Davies, who practices Transcendental Meditation, has conducted his own study to test the effect of group practice of the Transcendental Meditation and TM-Sidhi program on conflict resolution. His findings replicated several earlier studies showing a positive correlation between the number of people collectively practicing this technology in a society and the reduction of conflict throughout the entire population. His research also indicated a significant increase in the level of cooperation between opposing parties who were involved in conflict during the experimental period.

"The advantage of this approach to conflict resolution is that it doesn't require any intrusive intervention to resolve the conflict," Dr. Davies says. "It appears to make use of a fundamental level of interconnectedness among all members of the community to reduce stress and create coherence in the conflict area. The evidence is there that this approach warrants inclusion in any government's multilevel repertoire of concurrent approaches to promote the development and quality of life at every level—city, national, and international. It expands the range of tools for federal government. Leaders should be aware of it. They should be trying it."

The following charts represent a few of the more than 40 studies on the effects of the Transcendental Meditation and TM-Sidhi program on society.

Increased Positivity, Decreased Crime

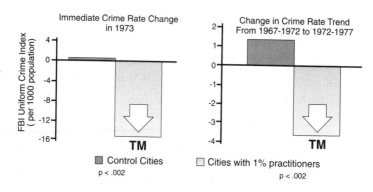

The results show that 24 cities in which 1% of the population had been instructed in the Transcendental Meditation program by 1972 displayed decreased crime rates during the next year (1973) and decreased crime rate trends during subsequent years (1972–1977) in comparison to 1967–1972, in contrast to control cities matched for geographic region, population, college population, and crime rate.

The Transcendental Meditation program and crime rate change in a sample of forty-eight cities, *Journal of Crime and Justice* 4: 25–45, 1981.

Improved Quality of Life

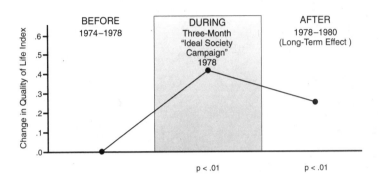

A prospective study was performed to assess the effects of the group practice of the Transcendental Meditation and TM-Sidhi program on the quality of life in Rhode Island. The number of TM-Sidhi program participants was sufficient to create the Maharishi Effect for the entire state. A time-series analysis was performed on a monthly index that assessed the quality of life in Rhode Island in comparison to a demographically matched control state. During the experimental period, an index comprised of the following variables significantly decreased: crime, motor vehicle fatalities, auto accidents, deaths, alcoholic beverage and cigarette consumption, unemployment, and pollution. In the figure above, an increase illustrates an improvement in the index of all these variables taken together.

Consciousness as a field: The Transcendental Meditation and TM-Sidhi program and changes in social indicators, *The Journal of Mind and Behavior* 8: 67–103, 1987.

137

Decreased Violent Fatalities

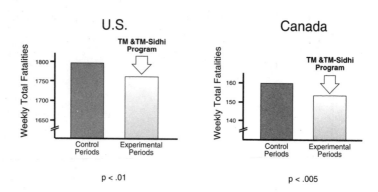

U.S.   Canada

p < .01   p < .005

Two studies using time-series impact assessment analysis found a significant reduction in weekly fatalities due to motor vehicle accidents, homicides, and suicides in the United States (1982–1985) and Canada (1983–1985) when the size of the groups practicing the Transcendental Meditation and TM-Sidhi program at Maharishi International University in Fairfield, Iowa, exceeded the square root of one percent of the U.S. population, or of the U.S. and Canadian population together for an effect seen in Canada. During periods when the size of the groups were smaller than the square root of one percent of the U.S. and Canadian populations, fatality rates were higher. The use of time series methodology ensures that these effects could not be due to random variation, seasonal cycles, or long-term trends in the two countries.

Test of a field theory of consciousness and social change: Time series analysis of participation in the TM-Sidhi program and reduction in violent death in the U.S. *Social Indicators Research* 22: 399–418, 1990.

Improved Quality of Life and Reduced Conflict

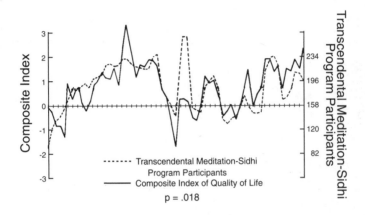

This study indicates that group practice of the Transcendental Meditation and TM-Sidhi program improved the quality of life in Israel as measured by improvement on an index comprising crime rate, traffic accidents, fires, and the number of war deaths in Lebanon, and by increases in the national stock market and improvements in national mood. The chart above shows the strong correspondence between the number of Transcendental Meditation-Sidhi program participants in the group in Jerusalem and a composite index of all the above variables.

International peace project in the Middle East: Effects of the Maharishi Technology of the Unified Field, *Journal of Conflict Resolution* 32: 776–812, 1988.

CHAPTER 8

The Next Step: How to Start

"**M**y wife, Jane, started Transcendental Meditation before me, and I saw changes in her right away," recalls Barry Pitt, president of a large retail business in Redford, a suburb of Detroit. "She was happier and much more outgoing. So I decided to learn, too."

That was 24 years ago—a year before Barry and Jane got married. At the time, Barry was a special education teacher in Detroit, teaching emotionally disturbed boys, 12 to 16 years old.

"It was a real stressful environment. My class was the last stop for those kids in the public school system. After that they went to Wayne County Juvenile Hall. Every morning when I would go to school, I would grab my keys, my wallet, and two aspirin. By noon I would have a splitting headache, and I would have to take the aspirin.

"The day I started meditating was the last time I ever took the aspirin. I never got headaches again."

Today, Barry runs a 25,000-square-foot hardware and automotive store with 120 employees. "A real pressure cooker," he says. All day Barry is talking with vendors about merchandise, attending meetings to set advertising and marketing programs, dealing with employees over personnel issues, and spending a lot of time on the floor working with customers.

Barry practices Transcendental Meditation twice a day. He says that it's part of his routine, like brushing his teeth or taking a shower. "It's essential. Physically, it keeps me strong, and mentally, it keeps me clear and alert. Because I meditate, I enjoy my life a lot."

In 1970 Jane Roman Pitt was a junior at the University of Michigan, studying education. She had heard about Transcendental Meditation from a friend, and when she saw a poster announcing an introductory lecture, she decided to attend. After the lecture she decided to start.

"At the time, I had been drinking about six cups of coffee a day just to keep going. I was in school and working full-time as a waitress. I learned Transcendental Meditation, and a few days later I didn't need the coffee anymore. And after I would meditate in the afternoon, I could study at night without falling asleep. It really made a difference. I felt much happier and more settled inside."

Today Jane is the mother of two teenagers: Jesse, 17, and Joanna, 14. She is also a composer whose works are performed by choirs and chamber groups around the country. Jane says the benefits of Transcendental Meditation are the same today as when she started 24 years ago—"only much more so. The only way I could handle all the roles and responsibilities that I have as a working mother—let alone enjoy them—is through the deep rest, energy, and mental clarity that I get from meditating twice a day."

People start Maharishi's Transcendental Meditation for a wide variety of reasons. Some may learn the technique at the recommendation of their doctor, to help treat a specific stress-related problem, such as high blood pressure. Others may be quite healthy but decide to start because they want to use more of their mental potential. Others may start Transcendental Meditation because they want to improve their relationships or help create a more peaceful society.

Regardless of the reasons one has to learn Transcendental Meditation, with the regular practice of the technique, all of the overall positive benefits to the mind, body, and behavior naturally develop. Transcendental Meditation is one procedure that simultaneously strengthens all aspects of life. It's like watering the root of a plant to nourish the entire plant in one simple stroke.

How Do You Learn It?

The Transcendental Meditation program is taught through a seven-step course of instruction offered through hundreds of Maharishi Vedic Universities and Schools throughout the United States and the world. (Please see page 191 for a listing.)

The course includes two lectures that provide the necessary intellectual understanding to start the technique, and four consecutive days of actual instruction—about 2 hours each day.

The course structure is as follows:

Step 1—An Introductory Lecture

The first step is a public lecture that provides an introduction to the Transcendental Meditation program and presents a vision of possibilities from practicing the technique. The lecture is about 90 minutes and includes:

• Description—what Transcendental Meditation is and what it is not.

• Benefits—the scientifically validated effects the technique has on improving mental potential, health, and social behavior, and on promoting world peace.

• How to start the technique—an outline of the seven-step course of instruction to learn Transcendental Meditation.

Step 2—Preparatory Lecture

The second step is also a public lecture, which provides an explanation of the mechanics of the Transcendental Meditation technique. It lasts about 90 minutes and includes a discussion of:

• How Transcendental Meditation works.

• Why Transcendental Meditation is easy to learn and effortless to practice.

• How Transcendental Meditation is unique and different from all other techniques of meditation or self-development.

• The origin of Transcendental Meditation.

Step 3—A Personal Interview

The third step, a personal interview with a trained

teacher of the Transcendental Meditation technique, provides an opportunity to ask any additional questions you might still have and to make an appointment for personal instruction. The interview takes about 15 minutes.

Step 4—Personal Instruction in Transcendental Meditation

The fourth step is the actual instruction in the Transcendental Meditation technique, which is held on a one-to-one basis with a qualified Transcendental Meditation teacher. In this step you'll actually learn to practice the technique. Personal instruction takes about 2 hours.

Step 5—First Day of Checking Seminar

The fifth step begins a 3-day series of 2-hour checking seminars following your personal instruction in Transcendental Meditation. This fifth step is held the day after personal instruction. It is to review the mechanics of the technique and to verify and validate the correctness of your practice. This seminar is attended by all the other people who received personal instruction the previous day.

Step 6—Second Day of Checking Seminar

The sixth step is held on the second day after your personal instruction. In this session you get the answer to any new questions you might have, verify the correctness of your Transcendental Meditation practice, and discuss the mechanics of stabilizing the benefits of Transcendental Meditation.

Step 7—Third Day of Checking Seminar

The seventh step is held on the third day after your personal instruction. Its purpose is to answer any new questions you might have, verify the correctness of your practice, and gain a vision of the goal of the Transcendental Meditation program—the development of full human potential in higher states of consciousness. The complete follow-up program is also outlined.

A Complete Follow-Up Program

Following these seven steps of Transcendental Meditation instruction, there is a complete, optional lifetime follow-up program that is available for every meditator. The program includes regular personal checking, advanced lectures and special seminars to ensure your complete understanding of the benefits. The seven steps, plus the follow-up program, are offered through Maharishi Vedic Universities and Schools located throughout the United States.

The Requirements to Learn

There are a few practical requirements to start the technique, including the time needed to learn the technique—2 hours a day over 4 consecutive days—and a course fee. For details on both, please attend a free introductory lecture on Transcendental Meditation in your area.

"This is a large university, and there are a lot of very competent people here, so you can easily feel that your work doesn't matter," says Joelle Tamraz, 21, a third-year social studies major at Harvard. "It takes a lot of belief in yourself, a lot of self-confidence. Some students fall by the wayside when they're not given positive reinforcement. It also takes an open and flexible mind and discipline and commitment to your work to be successful."

Joelle is an A student. She is considering an academic career or public service, after graduation. Joelle started Transcendental Meditation, along with her mother and sister, in New York City after she graduated from high school. She has been practicing the technique for the 3 years she has been at Harvard.

"After I meditate in the morning, I go to my classes and out into the world, and I feel confident and calm. I feel more prepared for the tasks at hand, which are often difficult and many.

"And although my studies are extremely important to me, since I have been meditating I feel that my life has a deeper sense of purpose. The experience of my inner self has allowed me to put what I do every day into a larger, more meaningful whole. As a result, my relationships with people have dramatically improved. I've developed much more loving and profound friendships, which I trace to the growing balance and peacefulness I have from Transcendental Meditation. And because I meditate regularly, I don't feel a lot of stress even when I have a lot of work. I am able to put things in perspective."

To other students facing the challenges of high school or college, Joelle strongly recommends Transcendental Meditation.

"It will give you a greater sense of stability and happiness and make you feel that you can easily tackle your day-to-day challenges."

Jack E. "Woody" Barnes, 47, an insurance salesman in Birmingham, Alabama, had always wanted to develop the potential of his mind. He had read a lot of books, heard a lot of tapes, and had a lot of different ideas.

"Then I decided to learn Transcendental Meditation, and finally I had a direct experience of what I had been looking for all these years—real expansion of consciousness. It's like driving down a road and suddenly the fog begins to clear. My mind is clearer now. I have experiences of unity in my life, whereas before unity was just a concept I had read about."

Woody started Transcendental Meditation along with his wife, Bobbie, an interior decorator, and his 17-year-old daughter, Frannie, a junior at Mountain Brook High School. The family has been practicing the technique for 6 months.

Bobbie: "I had bad hip pain. Whenever I drove for more than an hour, I had to stop and walk around. It had bothered me a lot for 2 years. My physical therapist said that a lot of the pain was due to stress. I remember one day after practicing Transcendental Meditation for a few weeks, I suddenly realized that the stress and the pain had completely gone away! And 6 months later it hasn't returned. My mind is a lot clearer and calmer now, too. And for me that's saying a lot. I am calm even when things around me are hectic. And because Frannie, who is my stepdaughter, and I sometimes practice the technique together, I think it has brought us a lot closer."

Frannie: "I love meditating. It's really relaxing. It's like taking a nap, except that your mind is awake, and you don't feel groggy or heavy afterward. It's very refreshing and gives me peace of mind. It has also helped me in school. I am able to cope with things better and I am able to remember more and concentrate better in my classes. Before I learned Transcendental Meditation, I used to get mostly B's, but now I get B-pluses and A's. Transcendental Meditation has also made it more peaceful around the house. There was always a lot of love in my family, but now there is a nicer, quieter atmosphere."

Woody: "Learning the technique has been wonderful. The teachers of Transcendental Meditation are great people, and the follow-up program has been absolutely outstanding."

After This Book—The Next Step

What do you do now, after reading this book, if you want more information about the technique? The next step is to attend an introductory lecture.

And if you have some questions about material covered in this book? Contact your local Maharishi Vedic University or School and speak to a Transcendental Meditation teacher. Or ask your questions at the introductory lecture. All Transcendental Meditation teachers have received extensive training—up to a year of study—to teach this very simple, yet very precise technique. They will be happy to answer all of your questions.

And just remember, Transcendental Meditation is easy for *everyone* to learn.

CHAPTER 9

Questions and Answers on the Technique

What does Transcendental Meditation do?

Maharishi's Transcendental Meditation provides the mind and body with a unique and profound state of restful alertness. The body gains an extraordinarily deep state of rest while the mind settles down to a state of inner calm and wakefulness. This process dissolves deeply rooted stress and tension, rejuvenates the entire system, infuses the mind with creativity and intelligence, and provides the basis for dynamic, successful activity.

I play tennis to relax. A friend of mine listens to music. Doesn't exercise or simple relaxation do the same thing as Transcendental Meditation?

Tennis, jogging, fishing, golf, gardening, reading a book, listening to soothing music, bowling, etc. are all relaxing, enjoyable activities. They provide a welcome change of pace, a break in the routine.

But the important question is: While they may

seem relaxing, do these activities actually release deeply rooted stress and tension? No.

This is because even though they may feel relaxing, nonetheless, they keep the mind and body engaged in some activity.

What is nature's antidote to stress? Deep rest—and the deeper the better. Transcendental Meditation is unique. It is not just another form of activity or recreation. Transcendental Meditation is a scientifically validated technique for providing the entire system with very deep rest—far deeper than ordinary eyes-closed rest or relaxation.

This deep rest has been shown to release accumulated stress and tension that nothing else comes close to eliminating—not a good night's sleep, a restful vacation, relaxation exercises, a great tennis match, or a stroll in the park.

Is Transcendental Meditation like hypnosis or other types of meditation techniques?

Transcendental Meditation is unique.

Hypnosis involves suggestion. Transcendental Meditation is natural and involves no suggestion.

All other forms of meditation or self development involve either concentration or contemplation. Transcendental Meditation is easy to learn, effortless to practice, and involves neither concentration nor contemplation.

Research comparing Transcendental Meditation with other meditation and relaxation techniques has found Transcendental Meditation to be far more effective for reducing anxiety, increasing self-actualization, improving psychological health, and reducing use of cigarettes, alcohol, and drugs.

Will Transcendental Meditation make me so relaxed that I won't be motivated for success?

Just the opposite. By eliminating stress and tension, and increasing energy and intelligence, Transcendental Meditation provides an effective basis for dynamism and success in life.

Transcendental Meditation is like pulling an arrow back on a bow. Draw the arrow back 2 feet, and the arrow flies forward 50 yards. Transcendental Meditation naturally draws the mind back to its own source, a reservoir of energy, creativity, and intelligence. After 20 minutes of the technique, you can plunge into activity refreshed and rested, with more creativity and intelligence.

The result: Do less and accomplish more with greater energy, success, and satisfaction in everything you do.

Can I learn Transcendental Meditation from a book or a tape?

No. Each person is unique; each person has a different nervous system and therefore a different pace of learning. Ensuring that you learn the technique properly requires personal instruction from a qualified Transcendental Meditation teacher. Reading a book or listening to a tape cannot provide the experience of pure consciousness and the corresponding profound state of restful alertness; nor can a book anticipate or answer all of the questions, at the right time, that every person might have while learning the practice. With proper personal instruction, you can enjoy the technique for the rest of your life—as well as all of the benefits it naturally unfolds.

Is Transcendental Meditation difficult to learn?

Transcendental Meditation is easy to learn and effortless to practice. Over one million Americans—and four million people worldwide—of every age (10 years and up), profession, education, and religion have learned Transcendental Meditation and enjoy its benefits.

When I start Transcendental Meditation do I have to join an organization?

No. Once you've learned Transcendental Meditation, you practice the technique on your own. There is, however, a complete, optional, lifetime follow-up program, available to all meditators, to ensure that they continue to practice Transcendental Meditation correctly and gain maximum benefits. You can take advantage of this program at your convenience.

Will my practice of Transcendental Meditation conflict with my religion?

No, it will enhance your religion. Millions of people of all religions—including clergy of all religions—practice Transcendental Meditation. They report that the technique, by increasing energy and intelligence and eliminating stress and fatigue, allows them to better follow the tenets of their religion. Transcendental Meditation is a technique, pure and simple. It involves no religion, belief, philosophy, or change in lifestyle.

Where do you meditate?

Transcendental Meditation is practiced sitting comfortably with the eyes closed for 20 minutes twice a day. It can be done anywhere—at home, in your office, on an airplane, on a camping trip. Anywhere.

How long does it take before I will notice some benefits?

It varies from individual to individual. All those who practice Transcendental Meditation do notice positive growth and development in their life; however, it's not really possible to predict what particular benefits you might receive from the practice or even how long it will take before you would experience a specific benefit.

Extensive scientific research and the experience of teaching the technique to more than four million people around the world do show that correct practice of Transcendental Meditation on a regular, twice-daily basis is very important for gaining the most from the technique.

And *everyone* can do it?

Yes. Anyone of any age, profession, education, religion, or culture. It doesn't matter if you believe in Transcendental Meditation or not. You can be 100 percent skeptical about the technique, and it will still work perfectly.

Transcendental Meditation is natural. It's just like gravity. If you don't believe in gravity, and you drop a tennis ball, the ball still falls. In the same way, Transcendental Meditation is automatic. It does not require any belief. It works for everyone.

And for those who think, "I could never sit still for 20 minutes," or "I'm too high strung, I could never relax," or "I'll probably be the first person in the world who won't be able to learn it...," don't worry. Everyone *can* learn to meditate. See for yourself.

APPENDIX A

Questions and Answers on the Scientific Research

Many people have questions about specific benefits of Maharishi's Transcendental Meditation. The following pages provide a more detailed discussion of the scientific research conducted on Transcendental Meditation. It gives you a concise reference guide to the benefits of the technique in the areas of mental potential, health, relationships, business, and society.

TRANSCENDENTAL MEDITATION AND EYES-CLOSED RESTING
Is there scientific evidence to show that Transcendental Meditation is different from just resting with your eyes closed?

Yes. Research shows that Transcendental Meditation is unique; it is much different from eyes-closed rest.

A comprehensive statistical "meta-analysis" was conducted that compared the findings of 31 physiological studies on Transcendental Meditation and on resting with eyes closed. (A meta-analysis is the preferred scientific procedure for drawing definitive conclusions from large bodies of research.) The study evaluated three key indicators of relaxation and found that Transcendental Meditation provides a far deeper state of relaxation than does simple eyes-closed rest. The research showed that breath rate and plasma lactate decrease, and basal skin resistance increases, significantly more during Transcendental Meditation than during eyes-closed rest. Interestingly, immediately prior to the Transcendental Meditation sessions, meditating subjects had lower levels of breath rate, plasma lactate, spontaneous skin conductance, and heart rate than did controls. This deeper level of relaxation before starting the practice suggests that reduced physiological stress through Transcendental Meditation is cumulative. (*American Psychologist* 42: 879–881, 1987.)

COMPARISON OF ALL TECHNIQUES
Are all meditation and relaxation techniques equally as effective as Transcendental Meditation?

No. All meditation and relaxation techniques are not the same. Four studies were conducted that compared findings of research on different meditation and relaxation techniques. These meta-analyses found that Transcendental Meditation is the most effective technique for reducing anxiety; increasing self-actualization; reducing alcohol, cigarette, and drug abuse; and improving psychological health.

• **Reduced anxiety**—A statistical meta-analysis of 146 previously conducted studies indicated that compared with every other meditation and relaxation technique tested to date, Transcendental Meditation is much more effective at reducing anxiety, the most common sign of psychological stress. (*Journal of Clinical Psychology* 45: 957–974, 1989.)

• **Increased self-actualization**—A second meta-analysis of 42 studies found that Transcendental Meditation was significantly more effective in increasing self-actualization than other meditation and relaxation techniques. (*Journal of Social Behavior and Personality*, 6, 189–247, 1991.)

• **Reduced substance abuse**—A third meta-analysis of 198 studies found that Transcendental Meditation was significantly more effective in reducing drug, alcohol, and cigarette abuse than were standard treatment and prevention programs, including relaxation. (*Alcoholism Treatment Quarterly* 11: 13–87, 1994.)

• **Improved psychological health**—A fourth meta-analysis of all relevant, previously conducted research—51 studies in all—showed that compared with every other meditation and relaxation technique tested to date, Transcendental Meditation is far more effective at enhancing psychological health and maturity. The studies showed that Transcendental Meditation promotes greater overall self-actualization, as indicated by increased self-regard, spontaneity, inner directedness, and capacity for warm interpersonal relations. (*Dissertation Abstracts International* 42(4): 1547, 1980.)

HYPERTENSION
Does Transcendental Meditation lower high blood pressure?

Yes. More than 30 million Americans suffer from high blood pressure, one of the most serious risk factors for heart disease. Sixteen studies have clearly demonstrated the positive effects of Transcendental Meditation on hypertension.

For example, a recent study was conducted on 128 inner-city, elderly African-Americans with hypertension. They were randomly assigned to either the Transcendental Meditation technique, progressive muscle relaxation, or a usual-care control group. All subjects followed the same diet and exercise regimen. After 3 months Transcendental Meditation produced an 11-point decrease in systolic blood pressure and a 6-point decrease in diastolic blood pressure, compared to untreated controls, and more than twice the reduction in blood pressure produced by progressive muscle relaxation. (*Personality, Elevated Blood Pressure, and Essential Hypertension,* Johnson, Gentry, and Julius (eds.). Hemisphere, Washington, D.C., 291–312, 1992.)

CHOLESTEROL
Does Transcendental Meditation reduce cholesterol levels?

Yes. Cholesterol is also a major risk factor in heart disease. A longitudinal study showed that cholesterol levels significantly decreased through Transcendental Meditation in hypercholesterolemic patients, compared to matched controls, over an 11-month period. (*Journal of Human Stress 5* (4): 24–27, 1979.)

REDUCED HEALTH CARE COSTS
Is there any evidence to show that Transcendental Meditation can lower health care costs?

Yes. Spiraling health care costs in the U.S. pose a dangerous threat to the health and financial well-being of individuals, institutions, and the government. The only permanent solution to the health care crisis is to make people healthier. Transcendental Meditation has been shown to be most effective in promoting health and reducing health care utilization and medical fees, compared to other wellness and health promotion programs.

• **Reduced health care utilization**—A large study of the insurance statistics of 2,000 Transcendental Meditation participants over a 5-year period gives an indication of what could happen if Transcendental Meditation were incorporated into existing health care programs. The study found that the Transcendental Meditation group had 50% less of the medical care utilization, both in-patient and out-patient, compared to controls matched for age, gender, and occupation. The Transcendental Meditation group had lower sickness rates in all categories of disease, including 87% less hospitalization for heart disease and 55% less for cancer. The difference between the Transcendental Meditation and non-Transcendental Meditation groups was greatest for individuals over 40 years of age. (*Psychosomatic Medicine* 4:, 493–507, 1987.)

• **Reduced health care expenses**—A study of 599 Transcendental Meditation participants in Quebec, Canada, found an average 12% reduction in medical expenses each year over a 3-year period. In the 3 years before starting the technique, the group's medical expenses had been equivalent to the norms for the same age and sex. Medical fees for "high-cost" individuals and older people decreased by 19% annually. (*Dissertation Abstracts International* 53(12:) 4219-A, 1993.)

AGING
What effect does Transcendental Meditation have on aging?

Successful aging is the best indication of how effectively an individual handles the stresses of life. Transcendental Meditation has proven highly effective in promoting successful aging.

• **Younger biological age (1)**—A study comparing people practicing Transcendental Meditation who were an average age of 50-years-old to matched controls on the Adult Growth Examination (a test measuring indicators of biological age: systolic blood pressure, auditory threshold, and near-point vision) found that the biological age of long-term participants in the Transcendental Meditation program was, on average, 12 years less than their actual chronological age. This means that a 50-year-old who has been practicing Transcendental Meditation for 5 years would, on average, have the biological age of a 38-year-old. (*International Journal of Neuroscience* 16: 53–58, 1982.)

• **Younger biological age (2)**—Higher levels of plasma dehydroepiandrosterone sulfate (DHEAS) is a hormonal marker of younger biological age. This hormone was found to be significantly higher for 326 adult Transcendental Meditation technique practitioners than for 972 age- and sex-matched controls. These differences were largest for the oldest age categories. (*Journal of Behavioral Medicine* 15(4): 327–341, 1992.)

163

• **Longer life**—Seventy-three residents of homes for the elderly (mean age 81 years) were randomly assigned to one of three treatments which were highly similar in external structure and expectation-fostering features: Transcendental Meditation, mindfulness training in active distinction making, and a relaxation program; while a fourth group received usual care. The Transcendental Meditation group improved significantly more than did all other groups on all the measures tested: systolic blood pressure, mental health, paired-associates learning, two measures of cognitive flexibility, self-ratings of behavioral flexibility and aging, and multiple indicators of treatment efficacy. Moreover, after 3 years the survival rate for Transcendental Meditation was 100%, compared to 65%, 77%, or 88% survival rates for the other treatment groups, respectively, and 63% for the untreated elderly. These results indicate that Transcendental Meditation promotes a longer life and a higher quality of life. (*Journal of Personality and Social Psychology* 57(6): 950–964, 1989.)

MENTAL HEALTH
Has there been research on the effects of Transcendental Meditation on mental health?

Yes. Transcendental Meditation has been found to improve mental health by reducing biochemical indicators of stress, decreasing anxiety, and enhancing psychological development.

• **Increased field independence**—A study of perception found that after 3 months those who learned Transcendental Meditation increased significantly more than did controls in their ability to perceive the world more accurately under potentially confusing conditions. Psychologists call this ability "field independence" because it indicates the growth of a stable internal frame of reference that makes the individual more self-sufficient and independent of the "field" of the physical and social environment. These individuals have broader comprehension and improved ability to focus and are better able to see another person's perspective, while remaining unswayed by social pressure to do something that they judge to be wrong. (*Perceptual and Motor Skills* 39: 1031–1034, 1974.)

• **Most effective technique to reduce anxiety**— As previously cited on page 159, a meta-analysis of 146 previously conducted studies on the effects on trait anxiety of Transcendental Meditation, other meditation techniques, and progressive relaxation and other relaxation techniques, found that Transcendental Meditation had a significantly greater effect on reducing anxiety than did all other treatments. This study controlled for a number of possible variables, including population, age, sex, experimental design, etc. (*Journal of Clinical Psychology* 45: 957–974, 1989.)

• **Most effective technique for enhancing psychological maturity**—As previously cited on page 160, a meta-analysis of 51 studies of different meditation techniques found a significantly larger effect from Transcendental Meditation, compared to other forms of meditation, on a wide range of psychological measures, including anxiety, depression, anger, self-esteem, and internal locus of control. The result was maintained in the studies of highest validity and strongest experimental design. (*Dissertation Abstracts International* 42(4): 1547, 1980.)

• **Less hospital admissions for psychiatric care**— The Swedish government's National Health Board conducted a nationwide epidemiological study that found that hospital admissions for psychiatric care were 150–200 times less common among the 35,000 people practicing Transcendental Meditation in Sweden, than for the population as a whole. (Suurkula, University of Gothenburg, Vasa Hospital, Gothenburg, Sweden, 1977.)

EDUCATION
Is there research on the effects of Transcendental Meditation in the schools?

Yes. Over 30 years of experience in schools, colleges, and universities in the U.S. and around the world, and extensive scientific research, have shown that Transcendental Meditation improves basic learning skills, increases intelligence, improves grades, and improves moral reasoning in students.

• **Improved basic learning skills**—A study of elementary school children found that students who practiced Transcendental Meditation over the course of an academic year significantly improved in mathematics, reading, language, and study skills. (*Education* 107: 49–54, 1986.)

• **Improved intellectual performance and self-concept in inner-city children**—A study of inner-city children found that through regular practice of the Transcendental Meditation technique, students increased in analytic intelligence, self-concept, and general intellectual ability. (Presented at the 98th annual meeting of the American Psychological Association, Washington, D.C., August 1990.)

• **Increased intelligence**—A study of college students who practiced Transcendental Meditation at Maharishi International University in Fairfield, Iowa, found that they improved significantly on a "culture-fair" (nonverbal) measure of IQ over a 2-year period, while no change in IQ was found in non-meditating college students from another Iowa university over the same period. Subjects' age, education level, level of interest in meditation, father's education level, and father's annual income were statistically controlled for in the study. No other procedure has consistently been found to increase general intelligence in college-age students. (Maharishi International University integrates the arts, sciences, and professions with the study and development of consciousness through the practice of Transcendental Meditation. The University is accredited to the Ph.D. level by the North Central Association of Schools and Colleges.) (*Personality and Individual Differences* 12: 1105–1116, 1991.)

BUSINESS
What effect does Transcendental Meditation have in a business?

Transcendental Meditation has been used in hundreds of businesses in the U.S. and around the world. Research in several business settings has found Transcendental Meditation to be a highly effective corporate development program.

• **Improved health and increased job performance**—Transcendental Meditation proved highly effective in reducing on-the-job stress and promoting employee health and development, when the technique was offered in the manufacturing plant of a large Fortune 100 company and in a smaller distribution sales company. The study found that managers and employees practicing Transcendental Meditation displayed less anxiety, job tension, insomnia, and fatigue, and reduced cigarette and hard liquor use, compared to non-meditating employees. The study also found the Transcendental Meditation group showed improved health and fewer health complaints, and enhanced effectiveness, job satisfaction, and work/personal relationships. (*Anxiety, Stress and Coping: International Journal* 6: 245–262, 1993.)

• **Increased job performance**—A second study found that Transcendental Meditation increased job productivity and satisfaction. In addition, relationships with both supervisors and co-workers improved. (*Academy of Management Journal* 17: 362–368, 1974.)

• **Case history of business success**—A 7-year case study of a chemical manufacturing company found dramatic increases in productivity and net income, and decreases in sick days, correlated with increases in the number of employees in the company practicing Transcendental Meditation. (*Enlightened Management: Building High Performance People.* Maharishi International University Press, Fairfield, Iowa, 1989.)

•**Improved health in Japanese industry**—The Japanese government's National Institute of Industrial Health, in a controlled longitudinal study with nearly 800 subjects in one of Japan's largest companies, found significant improvements in physiological and mental health in industrial workers who practiced Transcendental Meditation compared to controls. The meditators showed decreases in physical complaints, anxiety, depression, smoking, insomnia, digestive problems, neurotic tendencies, and psychosomatic problems. (*Japanese Journal of Public Health* 37(10): 729, 1990; *Japanese Journal of Industrial Health* 32(7): 177, 1990.)

TRAUMATIC STRESS
Has research been done on the effects of Transcendental Meditation on traumatic stress?

Yes. In a Vietnam veterans center, 18 men suffering from severe and apparently intractable post-traumatic stress syndrome were randomly assigned to either the

Transcendental Meditation technique or psychotherapy (multiple modalities). After 3 months of treatment, the counseling had no significant impact, but Transcendental Meditation reduced emotional numbness, alcohol abuse, insomnia, depression, anxiety, and severity of delayed stress syndrome. Veterans practicing Transcendental Meditation also showed significant improvement, compared to controls, in employment status. (*Journal of Counseling and Development* 64: 212–214, 1985.)

SUBSTANCE ABUSE
Has Transcendental Meditation been used to prevent and treat cigarette, drug, and alcohol abuse?

Yes. Cigarette smoking is the largest, non-genetic cause of death in the U.S. (400,000 people per year), and alcohol is the third largest cause of death (100,000 per year). Experts estimate that nearly 80% of crime is drug or alcohol related. Research has found Transcendental Meditation to be highly effective in both the treatment and prevention of substance abuse.

• **More effective than other programs**—As previously cited on page 159, a statistical meta-analysis of 198 studies, which compared all standard treatment and prevention programs for substance abuse (including Alcoholics Anonymous, individual counseling, educational programs, anti-smoking courses, anti-drug programs, and self-esteem training), found that Transcendental Meditation was far more effective than all these other approaches. (*Alcoholism Treatment Quarterly* 11: 13–87, 1994.)

• **81% quit or decreased cigarette smoking**—In a prospective study of 324 smoking adults—110 who started Transcendental Meditation and 224 matched controls who did not start—significantly more (51%) of the Transcendental Meditation participants quit smoking, compared to 21% for non-meditating controls. When reduction of smoking (at least five cigarettes less per day—a 25% average decrease) was considered along with cessation, 81% of the regular Transcendental Meditation participants quit or decreased smoking, compared to 33% for the non-meditating controls. (*Alcoholism Treatment Quarterly* 11: 219–236, 1994.)

• **65% abstinence rate in alcoholism treatment**— In a study funded by the National Institute of Alcohol Abuse and Alcoholism, 108 transient, chronic alcoholic patients were randomly assigned to learn Transcendental Meditation, standard drug counseling, or two other programs. Transcendental Meditation was significantly more effective than all other treatment programs. For example, after 18 months, 65% of the Transcendental Meditation group were abstinent, compared to 25% for standard drug counseling. (*Alcoholism Treatment Quarterly* 11: 185–218, 1994.)

• **89% reduction in use of illicit drugs**—An 18-month study of 115 high school- and college-age drug users in an out-patient drug rehabilitation center in

Germany showed that the Transcendental Meditation group had significantly greater reductions in drug usage and improvements in psychological health, compared to matched controls of comparable age, gender, and severity and type of drug consumption who received only standard out-patient drug counseling. After 4 months of Transcendental Meditation, drug use dropped 50%; after 18 months, 89%. (*Zeitschrift fur Klinische Psychologie* 7: 235–255, 1978.)

CRIMINAL REHABILITATION
Has Transcendental Meditation been used in prisons?

Yes, very successfully.

Currently, about 1.4 million Americans are behind bars, and experts agree that conventional approaches to rehabilitating prisoners have failed. In fact, nearly two-thirds of all inmates who are paroled return to prison within 3 years—often after committing further violent crimes. In the past 20 years, Transcendental Meditation has been taught to thousands of adult inmates in 18 U.S. correctional institutions and to hundreds of incarcerated juveniles in 8 U.S. facilities. It has also been used in prisons in 12 other countries. Research has found Transcendental Meditation to be very effective in rehabilitating offenders and reducing recidivism (the rate at which offenders return to prison).

• **33–38% reduction in recidivism**—In a study conducted by Harvard researchers of 133 maximum-security inmates, those who learned Transcendental Meditation decreased significantly in aggression and mental disorders, and increased markedly in psychological maturity, compared to matched controls and matched participants in four other treatment programs. Inmates practicing Transcendental Meditation also had recidivism rates 33–38% less than those of the four other treatment groups and the control group, over a 3 1/2 year period. (*Dissertation Abstracts International* 43(2): 539-B, 1982.)

• **35-40% reduction in recidivism**—In a 5-year study of 259 male felons in California who had been paroled from such prisons as Folsom and San Quentin, the Transcendental Meditation group had 35–40% less recidivism than did matched controls. Other programs, including vocational training, psychotherapy, and prison education, did not consistently reduce recidivism. (*Journal of Criminal Justice* 15: 211–230, 1987.)

• **Large-scale study in Senegal**—In Senegal, West Africa, in 1987, President Abdou Diouf introduced the Transcendental Meditation program into 31 prisons nationwide. More than 11,000 prisoners and 900 correctional officers learned the technique. Violence in the prisons decreased markedly and recidivism rates dropped from 90% to about 8%. The Director of Penitentiary Administration in Senegal Colonel Mamadou Diop credited the Transcendental Meditation program for the dramatic reduction in recidivism. (*Total Rehabilitation.* Maharishi Vedic University Press, in press.)

• **Comprehensive research review**—A narrative and quantitative review of research projects on Transcendental Meditation in eight correctional settings indicated that regular practice of Transcendental Meditation consistently leads to positive changes in health, personality development, and behavior, as well as lower recidivism, among inmates. (*International Journal of Comparative and Applied Criminal Justice* 11: 111–112, 1987.)

QUALITY OF LIFE
Is there evidence that people practicing Transcendental Meditation have a positive effect on society as a whole?

Yes. More than 40 studies have shown that group practice of Transcendental Meditation and the more advanced TM-Sidhi program reduces social stress, as indicated violence, crime, and international conflict in society and improves economic vitality and governmental efficiency. (For a discussion of the mechanics of this effect, please see Chapter 7, "Reducing Crime in Society and Creating World Peace.")

How did scientists measure this? To evaluate the potential impact of the Transcendental Meditation and TM-Sidhi program on society, researchers assessed many variables, including crime rate, violent fatalities (homicides, suicides, and motor vehicle fatalities), armed conflict, economic indicators, and broad quality-of-life indices, which include the above variables as well as rates of notifiable diseases, hospital admissions, infant mortality, divorce, cigarette and alcohol consumption, and GNP.

The results indicated that the effects for each of these variables, or for overall indices, consistently changed in the direction of improved quality of life when a sufficiently large group of people were practicing the Transcendental Meditation and TM-Sidhi program in society.

The following are summaries of four studies published in peer-reviewed scientific journals.

• **Decreased crime rate in 24 U.S. cities:** Twenty-four cities that reached 1% of their populations practicing the Transcendental Meditation program in 1972 were found to have significant reductions in crime trend during the 6-year experimental period from 1972–1977, compared to 24 control cities matched for total population, college population, and geographic region. Even when statistically controlling for specific demographic factors known to affect crime, such as median years of education, stability of residence, and pre-intervention crime rate, the crime trends in the 1% cities were still significantly lower. (*Crime and Justice* IV: 26–45, 1981.)

• **Decreased crime rate in 160 U.S. cities:** A study of a random sample of 160 U.S. cities found that increasing the numbers of Transcendental Meditation participants in the 160 cities over a 7-year period (1972–1978) was followed by reductions in crime rate. The study used data from the FBI Uniform Crime Index total and controlled for other variables known to affect crime. Causal analysis supported the hypothesis that Transcendental Meditation caused the reduction in crime. (*Journal of Mind and Behavior* 9: 457–486, 1989.)

• **Decreased crime rate in Washington, D.C.:** A study of weekly data from October 1981 through October 1983 found that increases in the size of a large group practicing the Transcendental Meditation and TM-Sidhi program in Washington, D.C., were followed by significant reductions in violent crime. Weekly violent crime totals in Washington decreased 11.8% during the 2-year period. Time series analysis verified that this decrease in crime could not have been due to changes in the percentage of the population who were of young-adult age, nor Neighborhood Watch programs nor changes in police polices or procedures. (*Journal of Mind and Behavior* 9: 457–486, 1989.)

• **Reduced armed conflict and improved quality of life in the Middle East:** This study found that increases in the size of a group of individuals in Jerusalem practicing the Transcendental Meditation and TM-Sidhi program had a statistically significant effect on improving the quality of life in Jerusalem (automobile accidents, fires, and crime) and the quality of life in Israel (crime, stock market, and national mood measured through news content analysis) and on reducing the war in Lebanon (war deaths of all factions and war intensity measured through news content analysis). The effects of holidays, temperature, weekends, and other forms of seasonality were explicitly controlled for and could not account for these results. As in many other studies, the pattern of results supported the hypothesis that the Transcendental Meditation and TM-Sidhi program group caused the reduction in armed conflict and the improvement in the quality of life. (*Journal of Conflict Resolution* 32: 776–812, 1988; *Journal of Conflict Resolution* 34: 756–768, 1990.)

The accuracy of the results of these and other studies was strengthened through the use of sophisticated methods, including:

- statistically controlling for a broad range of demographic variables, such as population density, median years of education, age, etc.;

- applying causal "cross-lagged analysis" methods, which indicated that increasing numbers of people practicing Transcendental Meditation is followed by corresponding improvements in society;

- employing "time-series analyses" to control for seasons, trends, drifts, and rival hypotheses, and to demonstrate temporal relationships among variables, supporting the hypothesis that Transcendental Meditation caused these beneficial changes;

- creating large groups of Transcendental Meditation and TM-Sidhi program participants in various populations to demonstrate positive changes on specific social indicators, such as crime, and predicting that these changes would occur.

Moreover, the results of the studies assessing the effect of group practice of the Transcendental Meditation and TM-Sidhi program on society are highly statistically significant. The probabilities that these positive effects could have been due to chance are very small.

Selected References on the Scientific Research on Transcendental Meditation

More than 500 research studies have been conducted on Transcendental Meditation by over 300 research scientists in 210 independent universities and research institutions in 33 countries during the past 25 years. The following are references for 82 selected research studies, all published in leading, peer-reviewed scientific journals.

These and other research papers have been compiled in *Scientific Research on Maharishi's Transcendental Meditation and TM-Sidhi Program, Collected Papers, Vols. 1–6* (4,400 pages). Reprints of individual research papers, as well as volumes of the *Collected Papers*, are available from the Institute of Science, Technology, and Public Policy at Maharishi International University, Fairfield, Iowa 52557.

PHYSIOLOGY
Metabolic, Biochemical, and Cardiovascular Changes

Physiological effects of Transcendental Meditation. *Science* 167: 1751–1754, 1970.

A wakeful hypometabolic physiologic state. *American Journal of Physiology* 221: 795–799, 1971.

The physiology of meditation. *Scientific American* 226: 84–90, 1972.

Autonomic stability and Transcendental Meditation. *Psychosomatic Medicine* 35: 341–349, 1973.

Adrenocortical activity during meditation. *Hormones and Behavior* 10(1): 54–60, 1978.

The Transcendental Meditation technique, adrenocortical activity, and implications for stress. *Experientia* 34: 618–619, 1978.

Redistribution of blood flow in acute hypometabolic behavior. *American Journal of Physiology* 235(1): R89–R92, 1978.

Sympathetic activity and Transcendental Meditation. *Journal of Neural Transmission* 44: 117–135, 1979.

Neurohumoral correlates of Transcendental Meditation. *Journal of Biomedicine* 1: 73–88, 1980.

Effects of the Transcendental Meditation technique on normal and Jendrassik reflex time. *Perceptual and Motor Skills* 50: 1103–1106, 1980.

Muscle and skin blood flow and metabolism during states of decreased activation. *Physiology and Behavior* 29(2): 343–348, 1982.

Breath suspension during the Transcendental Meditation technique. *Psychosomatic Medicine* 44(2): 133–153, 1982.

Electrophysiologic characteristics of respiratory suspension periods occurring during the practice of the Transcendental Meditation program. *Psychosomatic Medicine* 46(3): 267–276, 1984.

Hormonal control in a state of decreased activation: Potentiation of arginine vasopressin secretion. *Physiology and Behavior* 35: 591–595, 1985.

Long-term endocrinologic changes in subjects practicing the Transcendental Meditation and TM-Sidhi program. *Psychosomatic Medicine* 48(1/2): 59–65, 1986.

Physiological differences between Transcendental Meditation and rest. *American Psychologist* 42: 879–881, 1987.

The physiology of meditation: A review. A wakeful hypometabolic integrated response. *Neuroscience and Biobehavioral Reviews* 16: 415–424, 1992.

A neuroendocrine mechanism for the reduction of drug use and addictions by Transcendental Meditation. *Alcoholism Treatment Quarterly* 11: 89–117, 1994.

Electrophysiological and Electroencephalographic Changes

Spectral analysis of the EEG in meditation. *Electro-encephalography and Clinical Neurophysiology* 35: 143–151, 1973.

EEG analysis of spontaneous and induced states of consciousness. *Revue d'électroencéphalographie et de neurophysiologie clinique* 4: 445–453, 1974.

Theta bursts: An EEG pattern in normal subjects practicing the Transcendental Meditation technique. *Electroencephalography and Clinical Neurophysiology* 42: 397–405, 1977.

Short-term longitudinal effects of the Transcendental Meditation technique on EEG power and coherence. *International Journal of Neuroscience* 14: 147–151, 1981.

EEG phase coherence, pure consciousness, creativity, and TM-Sidhi experiences. *International Journal of Neuroscience* 13: 211–217, 1981.

Frontal EEG coherence, H-reflex recovery, concept learning, and the TM-Sidhi program. *International Journal of Neuroscience* 15: 151–157, 1981.

Participation in the Transcendental Meditation program and frontal EEG coherence during concept learning. *International Journal of Neuroscience* 29: 45–55, 1986.

Topographic EEG brain mapping during "Yogic Flying." *International Journal of Neuroscience* 38: 427–434, 1988.

Field model of consciousness: EEG coherence changes as indicators of field effects. *International Journal of Neuroscience* 54:1–12, 1990.

EEG Coherence and Power during Yogic Flying. *International Journal of Neuroscience* 54:1–12, 1990.

Health

Effect of Transcendental Meditation on serum cholesterol and blood pressure. *Journal of the Israel Medical Association* 95(1): 1–2, 1978.

Transcendental Meditation in the management of hypercholesterolemia. *Journal of Human Stress* 5(4): 24–27, 1979.

Systolic blood pressure and long-term practice of the Transcendental Meditation and TM-Sidhi program: Effects of TM on systolic blood pressure. *Psychosomatic Medicine* 45(1): 41–46, 1983.

Transcendental Meditation in the treatment of post-Vietnam adjustment. *Journal of Counseling and Development* 64: 212–215, 1985.

Medical care utilization and the Transcendental Meditation program. *Psychosomatic Medicine* 49(1): 493–507, 1987.

Transcendental Meditation, mindfulness, and longevity: An experimental study with the elderly. *Journal of Personality and Social Psychology* 57: 950–964, 1989.

Stress management in elderly blacks with hypertension. *Proceedings of the 2nd International Conference on Race, Ethnicity, and Health: Challenges in Diabetes and Hypertension*, Salvador, Brazil, July 1991.

In search of an optimal behavioral treatment for hypertension. *Personality, Elevated Blood Pressure, and Essential Hypertension*, Johnson, E.H.; Gentry, W.D.; and Julius, S. (eds.). Hemisphere, Washington, D.C., 291–312, 1992.

Aging

The effects of the Transcendental Meditation and TM-Sidhi program on the aging process. *International Journal of Neuroscience* 16: 53–58, 1982.

Elevated serum dehydroepiandrosterone sulfate levels in older practitioners of the Transcendental Meditation and TM-Sidhi program. *Journal of Behavioral Medicine* 15(4): 327–341, 1992.

PSYCHOLOGY
Creativity, Intelligence, Perception, Learning Ability, and Academic Performance

Influence of Transcendental Meditation upon autokinetic perception. *Perceptual and Motor Skills* 39: 1031–1034, 1974.

Increased intelligence and reduced neuroticism through the Transcendental Meditation program.

Findings previously published as "Meditation, neuroticism and intelligence: A follow-up" in *Gedrag: Tijdschrift voor Psychologie (Behavior: Journal of Psychology)* 3: 167–182, 1975.

Transcendental Meditation vs. pseudo-meditation on visual choice reaction time. *Perceptual and Motor Skills* 46: 726, 1978.

Creative thinking and the Transcendental Meditation technique. A version printed in *The Journal of Creative Behavior* 13(3): 169–180, 1979.

The Transcendental Meditation program in the college curriculum: A 4-year longitudinal study of effects on cognitive and affective functioning. *College Student Journal* 15(2): 140–146, 1981.

Meditation and flexibility of visual perception and verbal problem-solving. *Memory and Cognition* 10(3): 207–215, 1982.

Longitudinal effects of the Transcendental Meditation and TM-Sidhi program on cognitive ability and cognitive style. *Perceptual and Motor Skills* 62: 731–738, 1986.

School effectiveness: Achievement gains at the Maharishi School of the Age of Enlightenment. *Education* 107: 49–54, 1986.

Field independence of students at Maharishi School of the Age of Enlightenment and a Montessori school. *Perceptual and Motor Skills* 65: 613–614, 1987.

Transcendental Meditation and improved performance on intelligence-related measures: A longitudinal study. *Personality and Individual Differences* 12: 1105–1116, 1991.

Field independence and art achievement in meditating and nonmeditating college students. *Perceptual and Motor Skills* 75: 1171–1175, 1992.

Development of Personality

Influence of Transcendental Meditation on a measure of self-actualization. *Journal of Counseling Psychology* 19: 184–187, 1972.

Psychological research on the effects of the Transcendental Meditation technique on a number of personality variables. Findings previously published in Begripsvaliditeit van de NPV-Zelfwaarde-Ringsschaal. *Heymans Bulletins,* Psychologische Instituten R.U., Groningen, the Netherlands, NR: HB-74–147 Ex. See also *Gedrag: Tijdschrift voor Psychologie (Behavior: Journal of Psychology)* 4: 206–218, 1976.

Transcendental Meditation and social psychological attitudes. *The Journal of Psychology* 99: 121–127, 1978.

Effects of Transcendental Meditation on self-identity indices and personality. *British Journal of Psychology* 73: 57–68, 1982.

Kohlbergian cosmic perspective responses, EEG coherence, and the Transcendental Meditation and

TM-Sidhi program. *Journal of Moral Education* 12(3): 166–173, 1983.

Differential effects of relaxation techniques on trait anxiety: A meta-analysis. *Journal of Clinical Psychology* 45(6): 957–974, 1989.

Higher states of consciousness: Maharishi Mahesh Yogi's Vedic Psychology of Human Development. *The Journal of Mind and Behavior*, 10: 307–334, 1989.

Higher Stages of Human Development: Perspectives on Adult Growth. New York: Oxford University Press, 1990.

Transcendental Meditation, self actualization, and psychological health: A conceptual overview and statistical meta-analysis. *Journal of Social Behavior and Personality* 6(5): 189–247, 1991.

Transcendental Meditation. *Encyclopedia of Psychology* (2nd ed.). New York: Wiley Interscience, 1993.

SOCIOLOGY
Business and Productivity

Transcendental Meditation and productivity. *Academy of Management Journal* 17: 362–368, 1974.

Effects of Transcendental Meditation on health behavior of industrial workers. *Japanese Journal of Public Health* 37(10): 729, 1990.

Effects of Transcendental Meditation on mental health of industrial workers. *Japanese Journal of Industrial Health* 32(7): 177, 1990.

The effects of the Transcendental Meditation program on stress reduction, health, and employee development: A perspective study in two occupational settings. *Anxiety, Stress and Coping: International Journal* 6: 245–262, 1993.

Rehabilitation—
Drug, Alcohol, and Tobacco Abuse

The Transcendental Meditation program's effect on addictive behavior. *Addictive Behaviors* 5: 3–12, 1980.

The patterns of reduction of drug and alcohol use among Transcendental Meditation participants. *Bulletin of the Society of Psychologists in Addictive Behaviors* 2(1): 28–33, 1983.

The use of the Transcendental Meditation programme in the prevention of drug abuse and in the treatment of drug-addicted persons. *Bulletin on Narcotics* 40(1): 51–56, 1988.

Effectiveness of the Transcendental Meditation program in preventing and treating substance misuse: A review. *International Journal of the Addictions* 26: 293–325, 1991.

Self-Recovery: Treating Addictions Using Transcendental Meditation and Maharishi Ayur-Veda. New York: Haworth, 1993.

Treating and preventing alcohol, nicotine, and drug abuse through Transcendental Meditation: A review and statistical meta-analysis. *Alcoholism Treatment Quarterly* 11: 13–87, 1994.

The role of Transcendental Meditation technique in promoting smoking cessation: A longitudinal study. *Alcoholism Treatment Quarterly* 11: 219–236, 1994.

Rehabilitation—Prisons

The Transcendental Meditation program and rehabilitation at Folsom State Prison: A cross-validation study. *Criminal Justice and Behavior* 5 (1): 3–20, 1978.

The application of the Transcendental Meditation program to correction. *International Journal of Comparative and Applied Criminal Justice* 11(1): 111–132, 1987.

The Transcendental Meditation program and criminal recidivism in California. *Journal of Criminal Justice* 15: 211–230, 1987.

Family Life

Transcendental Meditation program and marital adjustment. *Psychological Reports* 51: 887–890, 1982.

Collective Consciousness

Change in the quality of life in Canada: Intervention studies of the effect of the Transcendental Meditation and TM-Sidhi program. *Psychological Reports* (in press).

The Transcendental Meditation program and crime rate change in a sample of forty-eight cities. *Journal of Crime and Justice* 4: 25–45, 1981.

Consciousness as a field: The Transcendental Meditation and TM-Sidhi program and changes in social indicators. *Journal of Mind and Behavior* 8(1): 67–104, 1987.

Test of a field model of consciousness and social change: The Transcendental Meditation and TM-Sidhi program and decreased urban crime. *Journal of Mind and Behavior* 9(4): 457–486, 1988.

International peace project in the Middle East: The effect of the Maharishi Technology of the Unified Field. *Journal of Conflict Resolution* 32(4): 776–812, 1988.

A multiple-input transfer function model of Okun's misery index: An empirical test of the Maharishi Effect. Paper presented at the Annual Meeting of the American Statistical Association, Washington, D.C., August 6–10, 1989. An abridged version of this paper appears in *Proceedings of the American Statistical Association, Business and Economics Statistics Section* (Alexandria, Virginia: American Statistical Association), 1989.

Test of a field theory of consciousness and social change: Time series analysis of participation in the TM-Sidhi program and reduction of violent death in the U.S. *Social Indicators Research* 22: 399–418, 1990.

Where to Call

For information about Transcendental Meditation, including the schedule of introductory lectures on the technique in your area, please contact your nearest Maharishi Vedic University or School. Maharishi Vedic Universities and Schools offer the knowledge of consciousness, bringing enlightenment and mastery over natural law to everyone.

Arizona
1110 N. 16th St.
Phoenix, AZ 85006
602 254-9404

Arkansas
21 S. College Ave.
Fayetteville, AR 72701
501 443-4013

California
2716 Derby St.
Berkeley, CA 94705
510 548-1144

2525 Charleston Rd.
Suite B
Mountain View, CA 94043
415 967-7242

3920 Williams Rd.
San Jose, CA 95117
408 247-8963

17310 Sunset Blvd.
Pacific Palisades, CA 90272
310 459-3522

10112 Fair Oaks Blvd.
Suite 4
Fair Oaks, CA 95628
916 961-0320

18632 E. 17th St.
Santa Ana, CA 92705
714 832-0328

3878 Old Town Ave.
Suite 200
San Diego, CA 92110
619 296-6565

Colorado
13650 E. Colfax Ave.
Aurora, CO 80011
303 360-7014

Connecticut
205 Whitney Ave.
New Haven, CT 06511
203 562-7000

Florida
2750 Spanish River Rd.
Boca Raton, FL 33432-8141
407 392-5418

1125 SW Second Ave.
Gainesville, FL 32601
904 338-1249

4525 S. Manhattan Ave.
Tampa, FL 33611
813 831-7979

Georgia
1750 Commerce Dr., NW
Atlanta, GA 30318
404 250-9560

Hawaii
Honolulu
808 988-2266

Illinois
Chicago
312 477-0102

Indiana
3434 N. Washington Blvd.
Indianapolis, IN 46205
317 923-2873

Iowa
Maharishi International
University
Fairfield, IA 52557
515 472-5031

Kansas
9303 West 75th St.
Suite 210
Overland Park, KS 66204
913 341-1888

Louisiana
7370 Airline Highway
Baton Rouge, LA 70805
504 355-6638

2411 Athania Parkway
Metairie, LA 70001
504 837-9642

Massachusetts
33 Garden St.
Cambridge, MA 02138
617 876-4581

Maryland
4818 Montgomery Lane
Bethesda, MD 20814
301 652-7002

Maine
575 Forest Ave.
Portland, ME 04103
207 774-1108

Michigan
231 Michigan Ave.
Detroit, MI 48226
313 965-0905

Minnesota
2700 University Ave.
St. Paul, MN 55114
612 641-0925

Nebraska
306 South 15th St.
Omaha, NE 68102
402 346-6656

New Hampshire
214 St. Anselm's Drive
Goffstown, NH 03045
603 644-0890

New Jersey
109 Valley Rd.
Montclair, NJ 07042
201 746-2120

1401 Ocean Ave.
Asbury Park, NJ 07712
908 776-6700

New York
12 West 21st St., 9th Floor
New York, NY 10010
212 645-0202

North Carolina
Raleigh
919 783-5544

Ohio
19474 Center Ridge Rd.
Rocky River, OH 44116
216 333-6700

Oklahoma
Oklahoma City
405 840-0108

1748 S. Carson
Tulsa, OK 74119
918 582-2564

Pennsylvania
234 S. 2nd St.
Philadelphia, PA 19103
215 732-8464

Rhode Island
141 Waterman St.
Providence, RI 02906
401 751-1518

South Dakota
4201 S. Minnesota Ave.
Sioux Falls, SD 57105
605 330-1940

Texas
5600 North Central Expwy.
Dallas, TX 75206
214 387-8686
214 821-8686

801 Calhoun St.
Houston, TX 77002
713 659-7002

Vermont
88 N. Prospect St.
Burlington, VT 05401
802 658-9119

Virginia
10801 Main St.
Fairfax City, VA 22030
703 273-6631

Washington
4317 Linden Ave. North
Seattle, WA 98103
206 547-7527

Wisconsin
23 N. Pinckney St.
Madison, WI 53711
608 255-4447

CANADA
National Office
500 Wilbrod St.
Ottawa, Ontario K1N 6N2
613 565-8774